ADVANCE PRAISE FOI
NEW EDITION OF *BODY* h~~ORROR~~

"An exploration of misogyny unlike any I've ever encountered, this reissued and updated volume brings us again into the excellence of Anne Elizabeth Moore's research and ability as a historian. She writes with wit, wry humor, and the instincts of a detective-novelist-cum-muckraking-journalist. In *Body Horror*, Moore brings us stories that will never leave us alone again."

— RIVA LEHRER, artist and author of
Golem Girl: A Memoir

"With lacerating wit and furious precision, Anne Elizabeth Moore connects the dots between labor, medicine, misogyny, and cultural production to reveal the scars and sores wrought by Western capitalism. In the six years since *Body Horror* was originally published, Moore's already-prescient writing now reflects the urgency, both personal and political, of upending the tidy narratives of a body politic that hurt more than they help. It's a necessary evisceration of institutions and imperatives that asks us to do something almost unthinkable: imagine better for ourselves and our communities."

— ANDI ZEISLER, author of *We Were Feminists Once:
From Riot Grrrl to CoverGirl®, the Buying and Selling
of a Political Movement*

"I laughed, I cried, I puked, I cheered. This visceral collection is one of the best things I've ever read—an essential, humane book."

— DANIEL KRAUS, coauthor of *The Living Dead*

"*Body Horror* is a strangely comforting book to read for its decidedly feminist, anti-capitalist, and anti-consumerist content. It is indeed a tiny bit horrific but written with a good dose of humor, and shows that, no, you are not alone in this cruel world."

— JULIE DOUCET, cartoonist and author of
Time Zone J

PRAISE FOR THE FIRST EDITION
OF *BODY HORROR*

"Sharp, shocking, and darkly funny, the essays in [*Body Horror*] . . . expose the twisted logic at the core of Western capitalism and our stunted understanding of both its violence and the illnesses it breeds. . . . Brainy and historically informed, this collection is less a rallying cry or a bitter diatribe than a series of irreverent and ruthlessly accurate jabs at a culture that is slowly devouring us."

—*PUBLISHERS WEEKLY*, starred review

"[D]evastating in its unwillingness to flinch . . . *Body Horror* is an incredible, touching, intelligent collection that looks beyond what's comfortable to examine what is true."

—*FOREWORD REVIEWS*

"By audaciously linking her disparate Body Horrors to a larger construct—more complex even than her own immune system, more menacing than mere patriarchy—Moore allows her essays, each plenty feisty in its own right, to punch significantly above their individual weight. Whether one is ready in real life to attribute everything from Crohn's disease to Pacific Time to the machinations of the market, Moore's arguments land with force enough to make even the marginally politicized reader think."

—*LOS ANGELES REVIEW OF BOOKS*

"Probing her own experiences with disease and healthcare, Anne Elizabeth Moore offers scalpel-sharp insight into the ways women's bodies are subject to unspeakable horrors under capitalism."

—*CHICAGO TRIBUNE*

"Moore herself is hyper-aware, and her unflinching worldview had the effect on me of a knife cutting through the wool pulled over my eyes."

—AUTOSTRADDLE

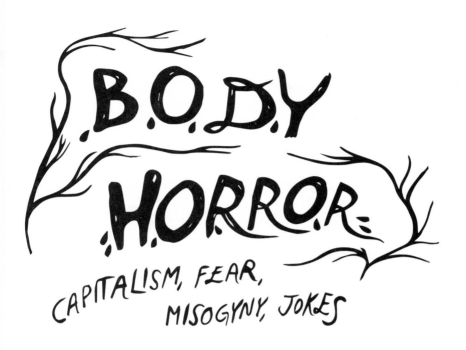

B.O.D.Y HORROR

CAPITALISM, FEAR, MISOGYNY, JOKES

ANNE ELIZABETH MOORE

THE FEMINIST PRESS
AT THE CITY UNIVERSITY OF NEW YORK
NEW YORK CITY

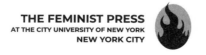

Published in 2023 by the Feminist Press
at the City University of New York
The Graduate Center
365 Fifth Avenue, Suite 5406
New York, NY 10016

feministpress.org

First Feminist Press edition 2023

Body Horror was originally published in 2017 by Curbside Splendor. The book has since been revised and expanded.

 This book is supported in part by an award from the National Endowment for the Arts.

 This book was made possible thanks to a grant from the New York State Council on the Arts with the support of Governor Kathy Hochul and the New York State Legislature.

Second printing September 2023

Cover design and interior illustrations by Xander Marro
Text design by Drew Stevens

Library of Congress Cataloging-in-Publication Data

Names: Moore, Anne Elizabeth, author.
Title: Body horror : capitalism, fear, misogyny, jokes / Anne Elizabeth
  Moore.
Description: First Feminist Press edition. | New York, NY : Feminist Press,
  2023. | Includes bibliographical references.
Identifiers: LCCN 2022056027 (print) | LCCN 2022056028 (ebook) | ISBN
  9781558612860 (paperback) | ISBN 9781558612976 (ebook)
Subjects: LCSH: Women—Social conditions—21st century. | Women—
  Health and hygiene. | Misogyny. | Capitalism—Social aspects.
Classification: LCC HQ1155 .M66 2023 (print) | LCC HQ1155 (ebook) | DDC
  305.409/05—dc23/eng/20221222
LC record available at https://lccn.loc.gov/2022056027
LC ebook record available at https://lccn.loc.gov/2022056028

PRINTED IN THE UNITED STATES OF AMERICA

CONTENTS

INTRODUCTION TO THE NEW EDITION

IN THE HALCYON DAYS surrounding the appearance of the first edition of *Body Horror: Capitalism, Fear, Misogyny, Jokes*, Christine Blasey Ford had not yet given testimony against Supreme Court justice then nominee Brett Kavanaugh regarding his sexual assault of her some decades prior, and he had not yet been appointed to the highest court in the land anyway. The subsequent wave of rape, assault, gaslighting, manipulating, undermining, silencing, controlling, and other revelations (ahem, "allegations") that we refer to as #MeToo had not yet occurred. There was nary a pandemic in sight. Banning books for acknowledging a panoply of gender identities was, if not unthinkable, at least uncommon. The gender pay gap was still closing, even if only by pennies every year. *Roe v. Wade* was still in effect. The sitting president, elected on a grab-'em-by-the-pussy platform, had not declared victory in an election he had clearly lost nor had he yet instigated an armed revolt on the Capitol.

It is difficult to believe that the first edition of *Body Horror* came out only five years ago. Half of that time has been lost to COVID-19, a constantly mutating virus holding sway over American health and culture that is taking a very long time for us to emerge from—will we ever? I have doubts—and that seems to be changing the nature of time itself. Deadlines have grown increasingly flexible in recent years, appointments now loosely held, memories

1

foggy. Could this book first have come out only five years ago? Or is five years an incredibly long time?

That *Body Horror* predicted and even responded to the above-named momentous cultural events was not lost on readers, and this appears to be one reason I still get regular emails about it, despite how difficult it has become to find copies of that first edition. Yet the book's prescience did not explain reader devotion, the intensity of which surprised me at first. This is a weird book: constructed loosely on seemingly unrelated themes, the text jumps wildly from location to location as well as from topic to topic, and I used a lot of what I think we can all agree is inappropriate humor. I genuinely did not expect readers to be able to connect with it. I had suspected for some time that when I became ill, I lost the ability to adhere to American Literary Logic. Most illness narratives in particular never made sense to me.

In constructing my own I did not, for example, want to share medical diagnoses, since mine are constantly shifting, which meant the volume couldn't be branded a Lupus Book or a Fibromyalgia Tale or whatever, and such branding, I am told, is essential to finding an audience. I was not interested in presenting a triumphal story of survival, since technically speaking I was sicker after the book came out than I was when I started writing it. My approach in this text additionally defies the dictum that readers want to think about illness only when they can feel uplifted by it, which strikes me as ludicrous. Plenty of people are entirely defeated by illness and also read. Are we not to acknowledge this reality? Even in nonfiction? Then again, I hold little interest in talking about my precise experience of illness very much at all, nor my favorite scenes from my favorite horror films, nor my experiments in femininity, sexuality, or, in any direct way, misogyny. I'm certainly no memoirist, as anyone who has read the memoir I published in 2021 can probably tell. More interesting to me is the collective anatomy, the public body, that corpus afflicted by our failures to protect public health. It seems to me impossible to address the frustrations of inhabiting my physical form without also acknowledging the difficulties facing other feminine bodies, other corpuses in general. That being said, I absolutely did not want to dump on capitalism for three hundred plus pages, even if our political economy sorely deserves it, because honestly that starts to get old quick.

What I originally wanted to do with *Body Horror* was take a few ideas, pile them up in the backyard, let them rot together for a few months, and see what I could get to sprout from them. Gender identity, gore, physicality, America. Somehow critics got it. Readers did too. I received emails telling me so after each new public reminder that the powers that be seem intent on destroying feminine physical forms. What a great thing: to get a kind email whenever a popular film director is accused of sexual assault, or my constitutional right to body autonomy is revoked by the Supreme Court.

But by then the book had disappeared. I mean it sold out, so another print run was ordered, and that one sold out too. Somewhere between the time the second printing was shipped to bookstores and when I should have started receiving royalty checks, the publisher vanished, and all hopes of keeping up with demand or getting paid disappeared with him. Many would cast this as the inevitable consequence of independent publishing, the predictable downside of working in a less overtly capitalist frame-work. But sorrowful headshaking in this case only serves the dominant political economy, reifies the status quo as just, fair, and correct. Will you be shocked to learn that I don't think it is?

So the first edition of *Body Horror* vanished amid a rising wave of women's voices responding to the loss of autonomy at the workplace, many also silenced or unpaid for their labor. Maybe this is the part that was inevitable. That a book about the horrors inflicted by labor, entertainment, and American healthcare on feminine and nonbinary bodies would disappear from the market just as it was becoming useful.

Books, however, are vital organisms, and I don't mean that they provide inspiration to human life-forms. Once published, they are living, breathing creatures of their own, with impulses, concerns, relationships, and a certain degree of autonomy in the world. Despite being born into what turned out to be a difficult, neglectful environment—both at its first publishing house and in that political moment—this one thrived. It found a chosen family. It developed new curiosities. When the opportunity arose to publish a new edition with the Feminist Press, *Body Horror* wanted to be something else.

I eliminated two essays entirely from the first edition: one about the superbug apocalypse because I did not want to have to spend every interview explaining the difference between a virus and a bacterium, and another about a horror movie I like about a carnivorous vagina and also a woman who wrote a bad book about vaginas. There were several good jokes in the latter essay, so I weighed this decision carefully, but the woman turned out to be an unhinged anti-vaxxer and no one ever saw the movie, even after I wrote about it, so I removed that essay. I also cut the introduction, which was an impressive piece of writing primarily for the number of words it utilized. I used some of these words, in their same basic order, in a new piece for this edition about fear and femininity called "Normative Bodies, Unusual Tastes." The remaining words are available for rent or purchase.

"Tips, Gags, and Jokes for Girls in Captivity" has been added to this edition, a piece written early in the pandemic and published by Pressing Concern Books as part of a series of bookmarks I made and mailed out to manage the stress of quarantine. The essay that directly addresses #MeToo, "Horror Autotoxicus," concerns the doings of a man who died a hundred years before anyone knew what a hashtag was, and "A Partial Recounting of My Current Anxieties" is, uhhhh—well, I'm going to let that one remain a surprise.

The rest of the book I revised, whether that meant recalculating statistics, adding new sentences, or entirely overhauling essays to more directly confront present-day concerns. "A Few Things I Have Learned about Illness in America," for example, has been updated to reflect several new things I have recently learned about illness in America. "Cultural Imperative," which in its original form was about the means by which the agency of folks with uteruses is regularly challenged by cultural forces, now includes mention of the overturn of *Roe v. Wade*.

As in the first edition, the essays in this book are ordered so that the reader moves from tangible, external, overtly politically charged space—the largest uprising in the history of the Cambodian labor movement, the gendered realm of intellectual property, the sudden vacuity of quarantine and the other isolating effects of illness—to internal, emotional, and therefore depoliticized space (in truth, the wellspring of politics). Symptoms, villains, and points of inspiration or joy appear, disappear, and reappear over the course of the book. Some of the essays are personal, but very few are intended to be personal essays; surprisingly little autobiography is contained herein, despite the number of people upset at how I portrayed them in the first edition, in which they absolutely did not appear.

This would be a good place to thank my editor, Lauren Rosemary Hook, publicist Jisu Kim, and the rest of the Feminist Press team; my wonderful agent, Sarah Bolling, and the entire Gernert Company; and the editor of the first edition of this book, Naomi Huffman. Various editors and friends helped shaped the pieces herein, including Lauren Kirchner, Daniel Kraus, Sarah Fan, Chris Lehmann, and Irma Nuñez Sless-Kitain, and I remain grateful for their input. For a bit, before this became something everyone did, I wrote a weirdo newsletter that shared a name with this project, the readers of which were generous and delightful and engaged and always offered screenfuls of hilarious, difficult, and heartfelt feedback that I still consult whenever necessary. I have recently acquired a horror-film-viewing partner, Jennifer Krasinski, and her endless enthusiasm for the schlockiest of gore makes me feel sane in a world that has lost its way. David T. Little, equally eager to talk about cats and cannibalism, deserves appreciation here. I must also thank my brilliant illustrator and beta reader, Xander Marro. We are all lucky to be living in a world in which she and Pippi Zornoza also reside.

I should further acknowledge that my approach to writing about illness as cultural phenomenon is profoundly indebted to Susan Sontag, and my devotion to doing it at all is because of Virginia Woolf. My thinking on women's rights and the best means to acquire them is due to a group of young women I lived with on the outskirts of Phnom Penh, Cambodia, in 2007 and 2008. The essay on Paul Ehrlich was completed in residence at Beloit College as the Lois and Willard Mackey Chair in Creative Writing. Kone Foundation and Write A House provided material support for the original creation of this book; its pandemic-era recasting is partially funded by the New York State Council on the Arts and is supported by a fellowship with the Ragdale Foundation and a residency at Yaddo.

The first edition of *Body Horror* was written to try something out. This edition is written just for you.

—Anne Elizabeth Moore
New York
October 2022

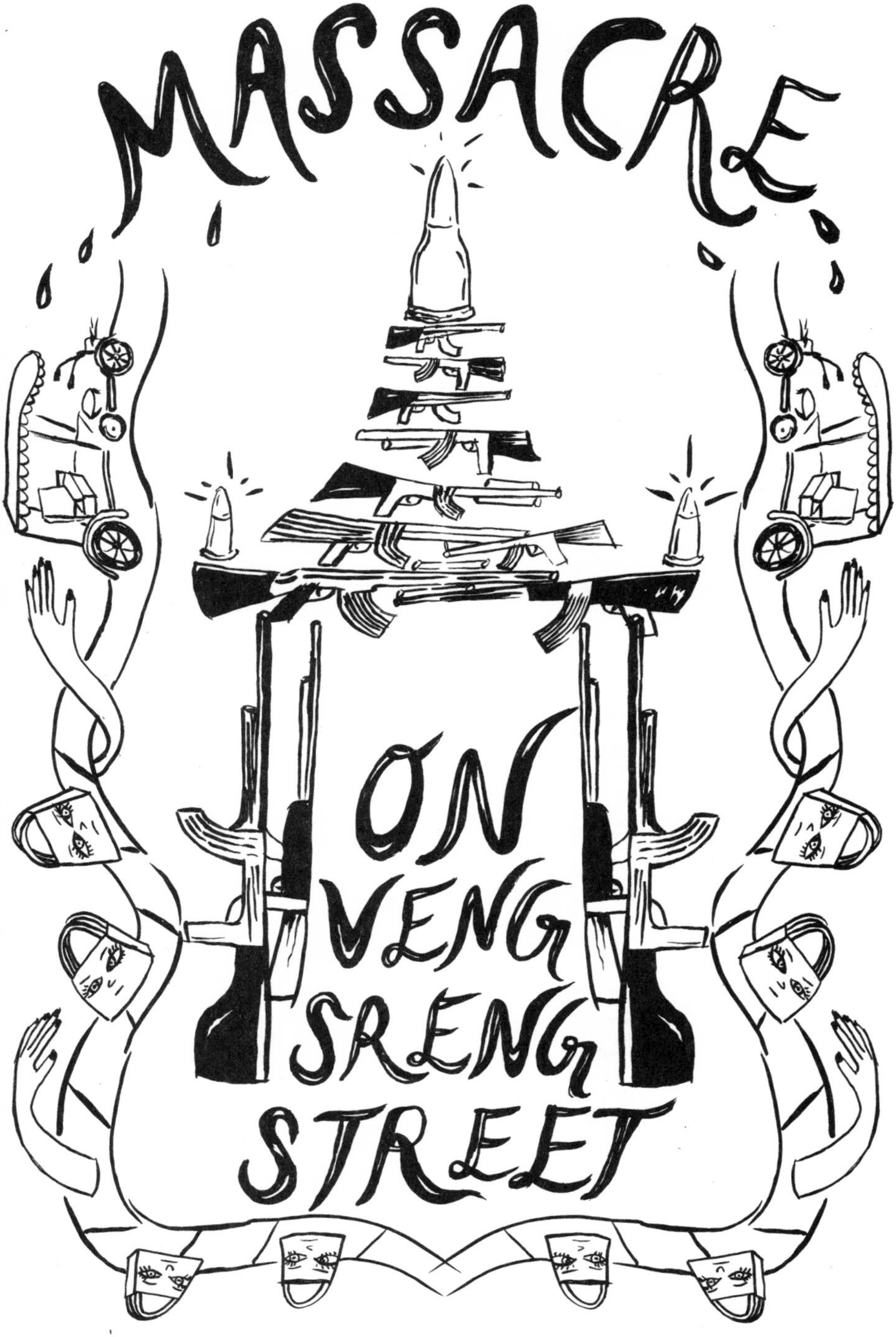
MASSACRE
ON VENG SRENG STREET

BY FAR THE MOST terrifying aspect of the grisly ordeal was that, four days later, everything had returned to normal. No evidence could be found that anything unusual had occurred. My nightmares started then—of adopting a charming baby that harbored evil intentions, of ordering a delicious-looking dish in a riverside restaurant that tasted of decaying newspaper, of strolling near a pretty pond that sucked me in, all allegories for an event I had experienced that started out friendly but turned dangerous fast. I rarely nightmare, so the midnight horrors were foreign, the fears of someone who's felt safe for a long time, but knew terror once: indications of joy gone horribly awry.

The second-most-terrifying aspect was that, five days before routines reemerged, Cambodians seemed cheerier, more open, and to be having more fun than I had ever seen. My experience in the country was limited to the seven years prior to 2014, but I witnessed thousands of people out in the streets at that time, beaming, brightly clothed, cheering themselves on for being together in public and openly proclaiming their needs. Travel brochures allege that the people of Cambodia are renowned for buoyancy and wide smiles, however arduously and famously long has run the nation's strife. Indeed, the Southeast Asian country's recent history includes periods of severe poverty, intense civil war, rule by the UN, a Vietnamese occupation, the Khmer Rouge regime, an unjustified

American bombing campaign, French colonization, and more periods of severe poverty—generations of desperate hunger and oppression only disrupted by a brief period of national independence from the mid-1950s to the 1960s when people still didn't have enough to eat, but felt proud and hopeful. Arguably, Cambodians were happier during the political demonstrations that started at the tail end of 2013 than they had been in almost half a century.

That was before the prime minister, baited by the opposition party, cracked down on the protests—the largest the country had ever seen—with machine guns. At least five were killed, more than forty injured, and twenty-three arrested on Veng Sreng Street in Phnom Penh on January 3, 2014. The next day, thugs hired by the ruling party moved into Freedom Park, the designated protest zone, and beat those who didn't immediately run for their lives while helicopters freshly donated by the Chinese buzzed overhead. The day after that, vigils were held while military police in riot gear and trucks ready to dispense razor wire dotted most street corners in the city center. The day after that, although a general strike had been rumored, garment-factory workers instead headed back to jobs or fled the city entirely, moving home to the provinces and accepting the poverty of rice farming when the possibility of getting gunned down by police under charge of a democratically elected government was the other option. And the day after *that* was Victory over Genocide Day, the day thirty-five years prior that Cambodia was invaded by the Vietnamese, who ousted the Khmer Rouge but then stayed to rule the country, which many remain angry about.

That was the day things went back to normal. The normal from before. When fear caused silence. When protests were disallowed, and gatherings of more than ten people in public spaces simply didn't happen. When people refused to talk politics. When no one accused anyone of murder, although everyone understood that murders had occurred.

♦ ♦ ♦

Freedom Park for me was like how people in the US talk about Occupy Wall Street. Of course, *occupy* means something different in countries that have seen—or admit to having seen—military occupations, so few in Cambodia had heard of the Occupy movement. My experience of Occupy Chicago was abrasive and sexist, but others found their politics there. *Everyone was so friendly! We were all in it together!* This was Freedom Park for me. Far more important, this was Freedom Park for the thousands of Cambodians who spent time there, most without a history of organized engagement to compare the experience to.

Each time I visited in December 2013 and the first days of January 2014 there were more people in Freedom Park, marchers from rallies and strikes corralled by Cambodia National Rescue Party (CNRP) leaders Sam Rainsy, Kem Sokha, and Mu Sochua. Newcomers arrived from the provinces, lured by pictures on Facebook, the social networking site of choice in the newly wired culture. People who didn't know each other made sure others had enough food, re-villaging the urban setting. Freedom Park was a park not in the Jens Jensen sense, but in the momentary-respite-from-the-roadway sense: a bricked slab with a few straggly trees here and there, to which occupiers tied tarps to create shade for themselves and whoever wandered by.

It seemed in all ways the opposite of the Khmer Rouge days, when city dwellers were forced into the provinces, food was hoarded when available at all, and neighbors couldn't be trusted not to report you. Freedom Park was beautiful and happy. Whatever may have felt unsettling for a moment dissipated quickly.

On my third visit, I was befriended by a newly arrived group of garment workers. I had been reporting on the Cambodian apparel industry for five years; garment workers liked me because I openly coveted their fashion sense, and tried to speak Khmer to them and failed. I acted like the girl who can't ever quite break into their cool group, which is exactly how I felt. A crew of six waved me over and gave me some peanuts; I ate them, although I am allergic.

I asked how long they'd been there. They told me three hours. I asked how long they would be on strike, and they explained, nearly in unison, "It depends on the GMAC [the Garment Manufacturers Association in Cambodia]." The government had announced, just that day, a wage increase to one hundred dollars per month. It was a concession to the protests that had greeted GMAC's wage-increase announcement a few days prior, to a mere ninety-five dollars. I asked if they were satisfied with the one-hundred-dollar figure. They were not.

"If the government does not give the salary of one hundred and sixty dollars, all the employees want to change the prime minister. They don't want him to lead again," one told me in response. Another repeated it, verbatim. It sounded canned. Several days later, after the $160 wage increase no longer seemed achievable, many garment workers would tell me that they didn't care about the government. They just wanted to be able to afford meat that wasn't rotten.

The $160 wage was a figure of some dispute. The CNRP had promised to raise the minimum wage for garment workers to $150 during their campaign, but when they lost the election in July 2013, the government announced a wage increase, floating $160 as a goal for 2018. The CNRP and unions began demanding it immediately, and rally participation soared. Rainsy, the bespectacled president of the CNRP, repeatedly told workers to fight for it, whatever the cost. He told them he would support them, and protect them, throughout their struggle. The government had a history of violently cracking down on protesters, shooting demonstrators, and striking garment workers with impunity. Sokha, the CNRP's second-in-command, announced onstage at Freedom Park one day that the workers were not afraid to die. (This turned out not to be true, but we wouldn't find that out for a few more days.)

In a photograph I took on January 1, 2014, the garment workers are flashing me a sign, raising seven fingers in the air. It is a reference to January 7, Victory over Genocide Day. The scuttlebutt I'd heard had a general strike planned for the sixth, leaving the seventh open to celebrate a day of renewal, the day the prime minister would step down, opening up the way for a true democracy in Cambodia. It's possible something darker was planned if the strikes didn't succeed; my Khmer was never that strong, and even if my tutor had taught me words for destructive activities, I'm certain the giggling garment-working ladies would never have said them to me.

♦ ♦ ♦

We'll call my translator and tuk-tuk driver Nike. It's a pseudonym I've chosen to protect him in case the Cambodian government reads this, but it's a faithful one: like his real nickname, it was chosen to signal the automatic respect and honor the nation craved, primarily available to the poverty-stricken masses by way of the brand names that passed through their hands, quickly and easily, in the garment factories.

Nike was attractive and lean, and raising two kids: a son he was educating and a daughter he'd sent off to live somewhere else; he didn't tell me where. On a tuk-tuk driver's salary (about $250 per month a couple of times per year, but $100 per month is more common, with occasional stretches when almost no money comes in at all), Nike could barely afford the bribes necessary to keep his son educated. Although the government is supposed to pay teachers, they often do not. When they do, it's very low (only fifty to seventy dollars per month for elementary school educators), so teachers request "thank-you money" from the kids' parents so they can eat. Going rates at Nike's son's school were only 1,000 riel per day, or about a quarter in US dollars, but $7.50 per month was more than Nike could afford. Education is not the only supposedly public service that actually requires substantial personal investment: they all do. It's what a nation awash in corruption looks like, and no amount of clever sloganeering by NGOs has curbed it. It is just how Cambodia works.

That's one of the reasons folks took to the streets at the end of 2013 and early 2014, before the massacre on Veng Sreng Street in Canadia Industrial Park, one of the country's Special Economic Zones. Corruption has kept steady pace with increasing cash flow into the country, and it's eating away people's chances for financial growth, or even stability. Corruption was not, however, the only reason—not, for example, why Nike was keeping a close eye on the protests since they started, nor why every morning began with his query about whether I had seen the latest developments "on Facebook."

Corruption hits some harder than others. It's a particular burden on women trying to survive on garment-industry wages, and most working women in the country are. Outside of garment work, there's not much an uneducated woman can do in a country with entrenched gender roles besides sex work, which (with Khmer customers) pays a little less than teachers' salaries before the bribes, or food vending, which pays about the same. A job at a grocery store or on the cleaning crew of a university pays about sixty dollars per month. If women can afford higher education, there's teaching—high school teachers can make twice as much as elementary school teachers—but Nike's already demonstrated how, with limited funds, educational opportunities for girls often suffer.

It is still worth noting that, even at $80 per month—the wage in place when the protests started in November 2013—garment workers made more than many in Cambodia. At the $100 wage, they would make more than most. And at $160, they would be among the highest-paid laborers in the country, as mostly women, and would remain one of the only workforces with a legally protected minimum wage. Perhaps most significantly, the wage increase would have been won by a popular uprising against the ruling party: a stunning display of political power.

That was never a likely scenario. The Khmer Rouge regime remains a recent memory for many, including the prime minister. Hun Sen was only a senior-level cadre in the regime before he worked in the Vietnamese government and then headed up the Cambodian People's Party (CPP) to win the first official general election in 1993. He's stayed in power ever since—partially due to his embrace of garment-industry money—so it was difficult to envision an outcome that included his agreement to double the current wage for garment workers.

Yet the arguments for a wage increase beyond any recent estimates of a living wage were compelling, if largely unvoiced. The population of Cambodia is around fifteen million, and the garment-industry labor force around four hundred thousand. As a body, these laborers are surprisingly influential: as the third-largest industry in the country, wages from garment work support the nation's second-largest industry, rice farming. If you distill this economic model down to a single countryside family, imagine how it might change mealtime dynamics when the girl no one could afford to educate five years ago becomes the family breadwinner. Her workplace needs grow vital to family sustenance. This effect, multiplied by four hundred thousand, is why garment workers were said to have been the driving force behind the sway toward the CNRP, the opposition party, in the July 2013 election.

Some suggest that this sway was larger than official election tallies showed: the results of that contest remain under dispute, which is another primary reason folks from all over the country gathered at Freedom Park toward the end of that year. Charges of ballot fixing and coercion at the polls plagued the CPP's declaration of victory, as they have plagued Hun Sen since his first election over two decades beforehand. In that time, he's led the country to the first economic prosperity it's ever seen. His nickname is Strongman, and a whole lot of murders, politically motivated and otherwise, can be linked to him. He's also one of the longest-serving leaders of any nation, a factoid that doesn't sit comfortably with those familiar with how democracies work. Yet Cambodians feel gratitude for whatever relief from abject poverty his policies have brought, and that is tough to overlook. Still, even official results—offered by the ruling party, natch—show that the CPP lost a record twenty-two parliamentary seats over the summer. The CNRP won twenty-six. The tide was clearly changing.

Yet the CNRP's Sam Rainsy is an ambiguous figure too. While many like him simply because he's not Hun Sen, he spent years in self-imposed exile in France, unengaged in significant political developments, including the fight for higher wages in the garment industry. He had helped to establish one of the most important apparel-worker unions in the country, although his dedication to workers lags in crucial moments. Many workers told me in near whispers that they wanted a change in government leadership, of course, but would be just as uncomfortable with Rainsy as prime minister as they were with Hun Sen.

▲ ▲ ▲

The day Varn Pov was arrested, Nike hardened.

Pov was the leader of IDEA, the Independent Democracy of Informal Economy Association, an ad hoc union for informal workers like tuk-tuk drivers, food vendors, and sex workers—someone I had met a few years prior, and respected, and I discovered was a friend of Nike's.

19

"How you know?" Nike demanded when I informed him of the arrest, his eyes getting big.

"Twitter," I told him. He used *Facebook* and *the internet* interchangeably, but hadn't yet embraced mobile micro-blogging. Nike folded his hands and leaned angrily on his tuk-tuk. "He a good man." He looked at me again and spit out a word in Khmer that I did not understand. Then, uncharacteristically, punched the back of the seat he'd been leaning on a moment before. He paced for a minute, and then said, "Okay. Now I take you to Freedom Park."

It was not a question posed deferentially, service provider to client: it was a command, a role reversal. I now offered him something more significant than cash for driving me places and translating Khmer: I offered him international eyeballs on what he could sense was about to happen in Cambodia.

He drove angrily, no longer chatty, for several minutes. Then he whipped out his phone—a dangerous, if common, distraction while driving a motorcycle, but he had things on his mind. When he got off the phone he shouted back at me, over his shoulder: "Anne. You know, I concerned about the human rights."

"You should be," I agreed.

The arrest of Pov and nine others on January 2 was the first retaliation the prime minister had taken against demonstrators calling for his resignation in 2014, but this was an old tactic of Hun Sen's that often preceded violence. In 1991, the CPP had over one hundred opposition party members killed while the UN ruled the country, Human Rights Watch has charged. Six years later, the prime minister's bodyguards led a grenade attack on a Rainsy-led rally. Sixteen died and over 150 were injured, shortly in advance of the general election.[1] Only months later, in 1998, hundreds of potential political enemies of Hun Sen's died or disappeared. After the results of that vote were announced, thousands of protesters swarmed the streets of the capital to demand a recount or new elections. Riot cops had cracked down then and cleared the protest site.

When Nike and I arrived at Freedom Park that day, we were greeted with chants of "Hun Sen must go," the rally cry of the moment.

Who cuts the tree?
Hun Sen
Who stayed in the pagoda and ate all the food?
Hun Sen
Who hurt the monks?
Hun Sen
Who killed the pop star?
Hun Sen
No more corruption
Hun Sen must go

The chant had emerged after a December 10 rally in Siem Reap. The allegations it lists against Hun Sen are so commonly understood as to be undisputed, and indeed, the prime minister himself acknowledged the lot once, laughing off the idea that he would resign over such trivialities. Illegal logging has flourished throughout the country; an activist threatening to expose it was killed by military police. The prime minister studied in the pagoda before ordering the dispersal of monk protests, over both land grabbing and, more recently, a Buddhist relic rumored to be stolen in revenge for an unpaid government salary. He also had an affair with a pop star who later turned up dead.

In a speech delivered that same day, Rainsy elaborated on the chant's allegations, with descriptions of how the Vietnamese were stealing jobs from hardworking Cambodians and comparing Hun Sen to a woman for refusing to take responsibility and step down. The xenophobia and misogyny caught him a few rebukes from human rights organizations, and another from within his own ranks by women's rights leader (and former parliament member) Mu Sochua. But xenophobia and misogyny can pull in support, too, especially when economic fears run rampant.

An elderly, toothless farmer in Freedom Park offered an example in conversation with Nike. He was from the Kandal province, southeast of the capital, and had been camping in Freedom Park for three days. "I want to change the government," he told Nike in Khmer. He wore a white shirt and a krama, the traditional Cambodian scarf, tied around his waist in a skirt, a style many city folk have abandoned.

"The government cut down the trees, stole the land from the people . . . and now they lost their relic of the Buddha," Nike interpreted for my tape recorder. The farmer could have been anywhere between sixty and eighty years old, and elaborated at some length on the forced evictions that have often preceded the development of land by CPP members or their cronies. But what he was really upset about, Nike translated, was that the Vietnamese held the contracts on the logging in the Kampong Speu province and many tourism sites in the country. Which was true.

To the farmer's left, a younger but somehow even more haggard-looking man broke in to explain something to

Nike. He went on for several minutes, uninterrupted, spitting as he spoke. The only words I understood were *Viet* and *Nam*, and when he ran out of vindictives, Nike translated the tirade succinctly: "He does not like Vietnam."

As we left the park that day, a song blasted through the area, bouncing off the street's metal roofs and lone, nearby skyscraper, heralding Sam Rainsy a national hero.

♦ ♦ ♦

I'm foreshadowing: I can't help myself. There was a sinister tinge to the air, although I was perfectly capable of overlooking it at the time. The truth is, thousands of happy young Cambodian women—smiles bigger than entire heads—were swarming the streets and the park, openly waving at me for the camera, chatting, hugging me, cheerfully declaring themselves political actors, agents of social change. During my first trip inside the garment factories in 2010, I gave a pseudonym to the factory to protect the workers and took no pictures of the women that agreed to talk to me; still I could convince only every fifth or sixth worker to tell me what she thought about her job. No one gave me a name. Tuk-tuk drivers would hush you in those days when you mentioned the prime minister, fearing that the wrong word in response would get them jailed or worse. Even the comparatively comfortable middle class resolutely shook heads, reminding me that change does not come overnight and that patience would be rewarded, before falling silent. An odd way to respond to the name of the prime minister.

In contrast, the visual that sticks with me from the earliest days of 2014 is a swarm of giggling young women,

23

dressed electrically. Cambodians joke that the way to tell a Khmer woman from a Vietnamese woman is that the Vietnamese woman likes to wear only one pattern at a time, paired with a solid color. Cambodian women like to wear many patterns, a mishmash of symbols and cute animals, clever if misspelled slogans in English, nearly incandescent colors. All together! As many as possible! She might wear a hot-pink top and bright-green hoodie with an American flag printed on the back with jeans, flowered socks, colorful shoes. They have plenty of time to concoct good outfits: they spend eight-hour days working in the factories where clothes are made, plus two hours of often mandatory overtime, and if they aren't able to afford or find a fell-off-the-truck version of something they like, a whole other batch of clothes eventually returns to them, cast-offs from the US and EU, cheaply sold in bulk in one of the city's many markets. More garments are discarded in the US every year as production rates increase, from 11.5 million tons of textile waste in 2005 to 16.1 million tons in 2015[2]—an ever-expanding volume of apparel that garment workers both create and look great in.

Perhaps because my pictures from that time are so filled with vibrant color, I can only describe being on the streets of Cambodia at the start of 2014 as the experience of pure joy.

🔺 🔺 🔺

Around 9:00 a.m. on January 3, workers gathered along Veng Sreng Street. Many were striking to demand the $160 wage, but some had other concerns: back pay at some nearby factories was still owed workers. The mood was light, however. One striking worker told me that, more or less, the protest was a big dance party.

Quietly, in the background, a military unit gathered. Later identified as Brigade 911, an Indonesian-trained force with an unruly history including participation in the 1998 election-related violence, they dressed in sparkling-new riot gear. They arrived by truck. They took out their guns, AK-47s and Norinco Type 97 Automatic assault rifles. Then, as a livid young man named Kha Sei told me in front of a clinic on Veng Sreng, "They fight the dancers."

Warning shots were fired over the heads of protesters. The crowd threw rocks and sticks in response. Police answered with live rounds, killing at least five, injuring and arresting many more. Several of the injured or arrested later claimed they weren't even protesting. One was a food vendor, working nearby, seeking to feed her family by selling food to protesters.

"When the police shoot the people, one guy died over there." Kha Sei pointed to a spot a few feet away. "He's still alive? The police shoot more."

"Were all five factory workers?" I asked. There had been no confirmation of this at the time, but Kha Sei, in his blood-red T-shirt, seemed to know all the players.

Sophy, a garment worker in her early twenties who was also there that day, crossed her arms and looked disgusted. A third friend, who didn't give his name, said yes. "But many more than five," this friend added. He pointed to a wall fifteen yards to our right, marking the property of Sun Well Shoes Co. "They throw one body there. Many others, they take away in the car." (Missing persons reports emerged later, although the official death toll was not raised.)

A striker standing near Kha Sei was shot. He mimed how he and two friends carried the gunshot victim to the medical clinic where we now stood, not thirty feet from where MPs were shooting, a point across the street Kha Sei pointed out to me. The clinic director turned them away. "He was scared about the government," Kha Sei said. The striker died. He stood over the spot, glaring angrily at the ground. I looked away out of respect.

Kha Sei spread his arm behind him, gesturing to the ruined clinic at our backs. "So we do this," he said. The building had been destroyed, gutted—everything smashable smashed, everything wrestable hurled to the ground and stomped on. The sign bearing the name of the clinic was riddled with holes, clearly caused by one young man on another's shoulders, one holding on while the other punched. The group chased out a woman who had just given birth, then tore through everything in sight.

Two days after the violence, the clinic was still a pile of rubble, testifying to a fury not released but delayed. The angry trio I interviewed stood at its entrance, glaring at everyone. The nameless friend's parting words to me were a comment that the garment workers were no longer demanding $160 per month.

"Now we just need machine guns," he said.

♠ ♠ ♠

Victory over Genocide Day was not the day of change the garment workers had signaled for my camera after all; it was instead the day Hun Sen held a special ceremony for a visiting Vietnamese delegation, to publicly thank them for their country's assistance in bringing an end to Cambodian bloodshed thirty-five years beforehand, even though a civil war continued to rage thereafter, and the bloodshed had continued. The bloodshed of recent days, too, went conspicuously unmentioned. It remains true to this day that the Vietnamese profit from tourism to genocide sites and Angkor Wat, the largest religious monument in the world, and Cambodia's beloved symbol of unity, strength, and pre–Khmer Rouge history. It is also still true that illegal logging hauls frequently end up in the possession of Vietnamese companies, and few investigations result. People remain angry about the post–Khmer Rouge occupation, and the extranational profiteering it allowed. Today, hostilities toward Vietnamese immigrants often result in violence or death.

Many garment workers had already left the city to return to the countryside, but those still in Phnom Penh on January 7 went back to work that day or the next. People fell into silence. Even Nike and I spoke less frequently. The country mourned, privately, each individual silently allowing hopes to dissipate, one by one. From the outside it may have appeared as if none of it had ever happened: Not the exhilaration. Not the horror. I might have ignored the whole grisly ordeal myself, if the nightmares hadn't started then.

But there was no ignoring it. In the earliest days of 2014, most Cambodians had taken to the streets in joy and hope for change. The government had turned on them, and many had died. The experience will never be forgotten, but it may never be publicly acknowledged either.

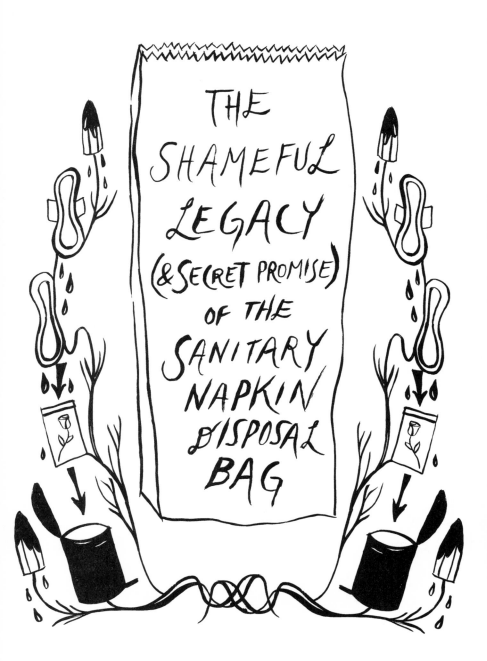

BY THE MID-1920S, the nascent menstrual-hygiene industry in the United States was in peril. Women, it seems, all aflutter about their recently acquired voting rights and whatnot, were persisting in the questionable activity of crafting sanitary products by hand. Following a tradition passed down by generations of matriarchs, panty liners were still being sewn from castaway fabrics—hence the phrase *on the rag*. This presented a massive barrier to the handful of companies eager to get into the menstrual-pad business. Who can blame these diligent entrepreneurs? They were missing out on valuable consumer dollars! So forward-thinking manufacturer Johnson & Johnson hired a team of efficiency experts to research the matter: Frank and Lillian Gilbreth, a husband-and-wife duo who combined their interests in industrial engineering with a study of psychology (and in their spare time, raised twelve children).

That the Gilbreths were offered the market research contract as a duo is significant because the Nineteenth Amendment was still new, and because they had a dozen kids, and because Frank died before the undertaking began. So Lillian was in a unique position to both innovate the field of market research—the Gilbreth firm was among the first of its kind—and to do so as a single woman. (The kids kept up the housework; their travails are immortalized in several *Cheaper by the Dozen* films.)

Hiring a woman for the job, even if the job was to look

into the habits of other women, was unheard of, although some saw Gilbreth's 1926 solo venture as a further expression of an emergent equality between the sexes. Johnson & Johnson, for its part, perhaps sensed that her status as a career woman and single mother might boost their own marketing efforts among that exact demographic. That Gilbreth was also in the process of inventing the field of industrial psychology—making her, at the time, the lone expert in the world on how consumers might feel about products, not to mention her ability to speak better even than her husband about the unique needs of menstrual-hygiene design—surely played a role in the company's progressive decision to allow her to honor the contract on her own.[1]

The company's problem was simple: catamenial bandages, as menstrual devices were called at the time, were underperforming on the consumer market. Gilbreth's guiding theory was that they did not adequately address the needs of menstruators. After all, Johnson & Johnson's main market competition was not other companies; it was the intended customer base, who had been fulfilling their own needs just fine, *thankyouverymuch*, for generations. Commercially available sanitary napkins were uniformly bulky, heavy, and uncomfortable, which Gilbreth set about proving in interviews with around a thousand women of diverse ages regarding their monthly needs. The resulting market research outlined a matrix of availability, adequate clothing protection, comfort, disposability, and inconspicuousness, all of which, when combined, would create a sort of menstrual-product magic that, it was hoped, ladies would be unable to resist. That, at least, is what Gilbreth's final report suggested, and Johnson & Johnson concurred.

Perceiving immediate salability in her ideas, the company generated patent after patent after patent based on her findings, quickly outpacing the production capabilities of other menstrual-hygiene-product makers, who strove to improve their own designs when Johnson & Johnson's new lines emerged just to stay in business.

In under a century, around seven thousand patents were issued for devices meant to keep menstrual blood in the pants area. These devices have become uniformly practical over time, ensuring comfort, leakage control, and disposability—and can even biodegrade, absorb foul odors, or remain entirely unnoticeable when worn and disposed of as advised. It is no hyperbole to claim that the bulk of these advancements are the result of one single woman's labor, nor would it tax the imagination to further credit the thousand or so other menstruators she tapped for input. Yet women's efforts go largely unacknowledged in the realm of intellectual property: the rights to profit from the menstrual-hygiene field—as assured by the US Patent and Trademark Office (USPTO)—remain with a group of inventors that is about 95 percent men.

▲ ▲ ▲

Equality between the sexes indeed.

One occasionally sees cited today that, over a century after achieving the right to vote in the US—theoretical though it may be in large parts of the country where voting rights are contested—women continue to make up 51 percent of the population but only 27.5 percent of the US Congress, and earn, on average, a mere 82 percent of what men do. (Factoring in race allows us to see that only white women can expect this comparatively high percentage of a masculine colleague's wages; Black women earn on average sixty-four cents per each man's dollar.) Implicit gender bias crystallizes in the realm of patents, for which women are listed on 13 percent of applications submitted globally. (On more than half of these applications, women inventors are paired with men; women are the solely named inventors on only 6 percent of applications.[2]) And this is just the application phase. At last count in 2016, women had been granted only 7.5 percent of total US patents, and an even smaller percentage of commercial patents were granted to women, just 5.5 percent.[3]

These trends have shifted slightly over time. A massive push prior to Y2K had women earning science, technology, engineering, and math (STEM) degrees twenty or thirty times more frequently than in years prior, and a change in patent holdings was one clear result: In 1977, 3.4 percent of all patents issued in the United States named at least one female inventor. By 2010, this percentage had grown to 18.8.[4]

The wage gap has shifted over time as well. It narrowed by approximately half a penny every year—until the 2010s, when it stagnated.[5] Women's participation across all patent-earning fields dropped during that same time period. Such stagnation is usually attributed to a mythological ambition gap between men and women. Women, it is often said, simply don't ask for what they want. However, this has been debunked by two different studies of the US labor force.[6] It turns out, women do ask for as many salary increases as men, but their requests are usually denied.

And that's even prepandemic. Many call it the economic

turmoil of COVID-19, but for a variety of reasons, women—particularly women of color—left jobs in record numbers after March 2020. According to the National Women's Law Center, over 2.3 million women have left jobs since the start of the pandemic.[7] Did they leave willingly to care for sick friends or family? Were they ill themselves? Unable to manage the stress of work as well as the stress of the pandemic? No longer willing to continue taking home a fraction of what men do, especially when going to work meant exposure to a deadly virus? Or perhaps they were simply fired for whatever reason seemed believable at the time. Likely some combination of the above, but the turmoil this causes even to our ability to track women's earnings is distressing: as women in middle- and lower-wage jobs leave positions, the average pay for women rises, and the gap appears to close. So even those eighty-two cents on the dollar should be viewed with suspicion.

Among the most persistent, trackable sites of gender disparity is patenting. In 2010, the National Women's Business Council discovered that the USPTO had record-high numbers of successful female applicants. Yet bias remains: "The ratio of successful women patent applicants to successful men patent applicants varies from a low 73.36% in 1986 to a high of 93.57% in 2002," the report states.[8] Somewhere between those two figures lies the true number of women who applied for but were denied patents on the basis of gender.

It gets worse. A 2018 report found that women inventors were denied applications more frequently and appeals to their rejections were mounted less often. Too, patents granted women had fewer original claims allowed than patents granted men—meaning their scope and value were restricted during the application process—and these patents were allowed to lapse more frequently.[9]

▲ ▲ ▲

Gilbreth's dedication to ensuring access to menstrual products that people might actually use allowed the sanitary-napkin industry to survive and soon thrive. The field quickly grew to offer a stunning variety of contraptions and palliatives, all intended to further mask the menstrual cycle as women entered, and then gained standing in, a workforce dominated by men. Noting that no concurrent moves have been made to socially normalize the regular occurrence of menstruation (the notion that Hillary Clinton might use a restroom for any purpose whatsoever was enough to set off opposing presidential candidate Donald Trump after one 2016 debate, for example) may spark the realization that the entire sanitary-product industry exists to allow menstruators to pass through an arena dominated by cis men without raising alarm. (Continue on this thought trajectory for too long, however, and you'll discover that far more effort has gone into the innovation of menstrual pads than into the establishment of women's rights, which is a line of thought I do not advise for those who already suffer from depression.)

Devices new to the market in the last century or so therefore vary in both considerateness and usefulness. Absorbent underpants, one might argue, offer little that menstrual pads don't, although other recent inventions are slightly more innovative. Tampons—absorbent insertables intended to soak up menstrual blood—take some adjusting to, as does the menstrual cup, another form of insertable that pretty much does what it says on the tin. Each carries potential hazards that range from embarrassing to life-threatening, but all allow for unimpeded movement with little blood overflow. (Unless you're on a heavy day and you sneeze.) Douches, on the other hand, intended to eliminate certain smells, come with fairly serious health hazards. They temporarily wipe out odor-creating bacteria, but also eliminate odor-eating bacteria, subsequently killing off your body's ability to regulate its own smell or, more dangerously, fight infection. Other sprays, ointments, and geegaws abound, each purporting to serve the basic purpose of masking half the world's natural bodily processes from the other half. Not to get too twelve-year-old boy about it, but it's difficult not to burst out laughing at the ridiculous products those of us who menstruate are urged to make use of just to experience the pleasure of going outside.

One standout product in the menstrual-hygiene field is the lowly sanitary napkin disposal bag. It is possible that you have never seen one, so let me describe them for you. First and foremost, they are bags, a fact central to their oft-mocked status. Usually paper, although occasionally plastic, they are intended to house soiled sanitary products, shielding contents from view of other restroom users. They have no other intended purpose. Because you are extremely unlikely to require them in the privacy of your own home, such bags are found most frequently inside the stalls of public restrooms, although never on the shelves of your local drugstore.

Basically fancified scraps of paper to wrap waste in, the devices come heavily decorated. Sanitary napkin disposal bags may be decorated with happy, willowy figures engaged in playful activities, such as tennis or dancing, or festooned with gay flowers. Some may feature a stick figure in a dress delightfully throwing an object into the garbage. Others recall a traditional—frequently Victorian—notion of femininity, and thus convey decorum. (The ad copy for a stainless-steel garbage receptacle, into which such a bag is meant to be placed, similarly claims it "adds a touch of class to any restroom.") Class-striving discretion is important—these bags do hold a specific kind of very dirty garbage from which other garbage, presumably, must be protected—but on the whole, sanitary napkin disposal bags strive to express ease of use, tranquility of mind, or maybe even "fun."

The bags' lighthearted design schemes contrast starkly with manufacturers' overt marketing strategies. These can be found on product descriptions in office-supply catalogs, promotional copy intended for the purchaser rather than the user. Sanitary napkin disposal bag producer Scensibles, in the section of its website labeled The Solution, lists a myriad of problems facing all who enter women's restrooms: microbes, smells, spillage, needles, and blocked plumbing—all, somehow, removed by the addition of a branded receptacle for pink plastic bags. An apparently short-lived website in 2014 called Teens'n'Parents went a step further: "Disposal of Sanitary napkin is the major problem polluting the environment [*sic*]." (Not offered for comparison was the pollutive output from sanitary-napkin manufacturing plants.) The nicknames used when the products appear in books and films and on shows or podcasts are no less alarming: sani-bag, individual feminine hygiene receptacle, lady bag, and even vagina bag.

The alternating intents of the design and marketing

teams for these products is fascinating. While ads intend to browbeat the purchaser into addressing The Problem of seeping uterine juice with a hefty order of sanitary napkin disposal bags, the product itself goes out of its way to assure users that they are behaving correctly, without effort, and possibly even enjoying themselves. One suspects that the bifurcated messaging is no accident, merely gendered for perceived audiences. Case in point: a trade mag op-ed by Scensibles founder Ann Germanow pits the issue as plumbers (95 percent men, nationally) and company bill payers (CEOs of Fortune 500 companies, as an example, are 98 percent men) versus tampon users, coded here exclusively as women.[10] (That biology and gender do not faithfully align has apparently not yet occurred to the sanitary napkin disposal bag community.) "A recent janitorial services blog confirms that if no acceptable alternative for disposal is offered, women ignore the signage and flush anyway," Germanow states authoritatively.

Certainly, the message embedded in the product's very existence is as gendered as the restrooms in which the bags are most often found, a wordless reminder to all who identify as women that the monthly waste of menstruators must be prebagged, a clear indication that it is more disgusting than all other forms of waste combined. "The number-one bacteria hot spot in a woman's restroom is the 'sanitary' napkin disposal unit," Germanow contends in her op-ed. Perhaps that tiny, classy waste container can more properly be viewed as a breeding ground for neoliberal subjectivity, a stealthy mixture of individually targeted fortitude and self-doubt that can be assuaged only by the relentless purchase of beauty products. If the impact of these bags on the psyche seems brutal, however, let's pause to reflect on their impact on the planet. The paper waste, plastics, and manufacturing by-products created will surely fail to decompose over the course of several more lifetimes.

At first glance, the individualized menstrual-hygiene-waste receptacle appears ridiculous. On closer inspection it may just horrify.

♦ ♦ ♦

All told, little good can be said about sanitary napkin disposal bags. That is, unless you care about gender equality. For these tiny, decorative gore-encasement devices do more than any other product in the field of menstrual hygiene to eliminate the earning gap between men and women.

Around four thousand patents include the phrase *feminine product disposal*, but very few of these have been awarded for bags created to house soiled hygiene items. In sum, close to fifty patents have been granted for sanitary napkin disposal bags—each, legally speaking, a unique approach to personal containers intended to whisk menstrual waste away from public view. Considering that they really are only *bags*, let's keep in mind, it should perhaps astound that close to fifty different patents have been awarded for innovating methods of placing unseemly waste inside a container before it goes into a larger receptacle for regular garbage disposal.

In truth, receptacles intended for the exclusive disposal of used sanitary napkins are made largely unnecessary by Gilbreth's extensive efforts. Menstrual products today continue to be self-contained, unnoticeable, and spill proof, as per her 1926 recommendations and the subsequent slew of patents that arose from them. Most restroom stalls do come equipped with small trash containers for such waste, which could, in a worst-case scenario, be wrapped in paper, conveniently located in the immediate vicinity of toilets throughout most of the Western world. If a small trash container, or any toilet paper, is for some reason absent from each individual stall, most likely there will still be a trash container in the restroom proper. In a worst-case scenario, it is true, in a public restroom, other restroom users may see you and be forced to acknowledge that you menstruate, which they may also do on a regular basis (and if they do not, they will certainly not be surprised that you do). Defenders of the sanitary napkin disposal bag—manufacturers, plumbers, and building owners, for the most part, with whom I have engaged in spirited online conversation—tell us that the primary purpose of such bags is to remind women that sanitary products are not to be flushed down the toilet. How shockingly inefficient! A sign in a stall would do just as well, or eliminating the potential for more paper waste entirely: include plumbing lessons in home economics courses at the middle school level.

Sustained consideration will lead you to wonder whether sanitary napkin disposal bags might not be capitalism's ideal form: an environmentally and emotionally destructive, eminently saleable, necessarily disposable, and cheaply manufactured good with little to no unique functional value around which a dedicated audience can be manufactured and endless profits derived therefrom. All part and parcel of a larger project, to mask the natural bodily processes of half the population. They are truly exemplary, these menstrual-hygiene products; all the more so for being such a humble—even, dare I say, useless—invention.

However fully the bags themselves perform and entrench misogyny, however, their design and manufacture promise a gender-equitable future: of the approximately fifty patents for feminine hygiene personal-sized waste containers, 26 percent are owned by men, 30 percent are owned by teams including at least one man and at least one woman, and 44 percent are owned by women inventors alone.[11] To get more specific, patents on bags that protect trash from truly offensive menstrual garbage are owned by a staggering 59 percent female inventors.

It is where capitalism gets interesting. Because the profits into which sanitary napkin disposal bags are eating are not those of the 2 percent of women CEOs of Fortune 500 companies, nor are sani-bags being purchased with the eighty-two cents that women are taking home for each male coworker's dollar. A predominantly masculine economy, driven by a fear of menstrual blood, is funding a pool of nearly 60 percent female inventors.

Lillian Gilbreth would certainly have been proud. Gender equity is finally within reach! The question we must ask ourselves, close to a century since her efforts— not to overlook the uncredited labor of thousands of other women—saved the flailing feminine-hygiene industry, is whether we want it under these conditions.

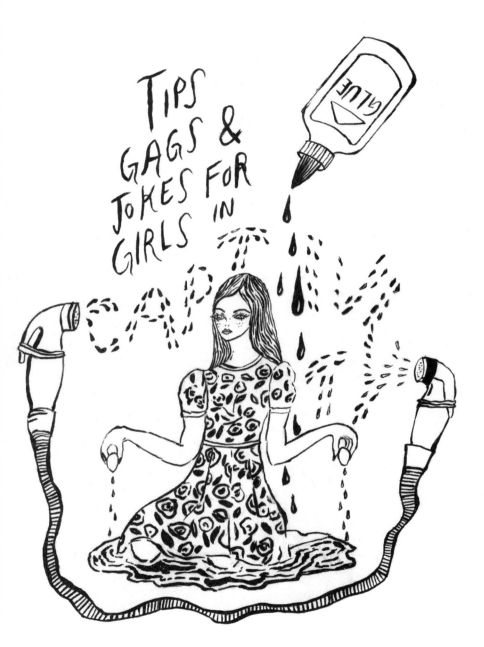

THERE ARE PLENTY OF reasons nowadays why a girl might find herself, say, unable to access human contact, engage in normal business activities, participate in a conversation without the aid of technology, or enter a building that she does not also work, rest, and play in. Global health crisis is a popular one, although there are others. Maybe sudden-onset extreme sunlight allergy. Perhaps you have fallen into a well, or an errant bottle of strong adhesive unleashed itself in your bed while you slept. That would do it. Certain apocalypses too. Situations of domestic violence are not uncommon; statistics show a surprisingly large number of girls also seem to find themselves human trafficked.

A man walks into a bar. Bartender goes, "What are you doing, we've been closed for six months, why aren't you wearing a mask, if you really need a drink you can visit our online store and order a cocktail for curbside pickup."

The precise details of your captivity are, for the moment, inconsequential, and best left to be sorted by the fire department, your family or friends, the vengeful stalker that's been obsessed with you for seventeen years, human rights organizations, or an international war crime tribunal. Our task for the moment is to focus on your day-to-day. As a friend who was kidnapped by the FARC for a year once said, "Don't talk politics at the dinner table." What he meant was: a girl's gotta eat.

There once was a man from Nantucket. Nantucket has had no new cases in six days. Why would he leave? But it's too late. He can't go back now without a two-week quarantine, and even after that there's constant testing, contact tracing. That town has a standard to maintain. It might be best for him to stay away so case numbers remain low.

What matters about life in captivity is that you neither have a choice about it nor a timeline. You may feel out of control, even though it is your own life. You are! Although this is also true when you are in the state that you now remember as free. Yet whatever degree of freedom you feel you can access in your regular life is further limited in captivity, and this may make you angry. Indeed it should. One frustration you are sure to encounter is that however angry you may become, you still remain in captivity. That you still have to live with yourself, and perhaps only yourself, suggests that it may be best at this time to set aside your anger. It is almost guaranteed to still be there when you can do something about it.

How many COVID-19 patients does it take to change a light bulb? Hopefully only one because fuck if I am going to help them out.

Once you set aside your anger and concentrate on you, you may find yourself, as a lot of girls in your situation do, intolerably bored. This is extremely common, and happens for any number of reasons. Perhaps you had a happy childhood and never learned how to cultivate the active inner life the rest of us get by on. That must have been hard. Or maybe you neglected to properly pack a bag with water-color paints, a smartphone, sourdough starter, and a copy of *Infinite Jest* before finding yourself at the bottom of that well. Next time you'll know better. Possibly you have just spent too long cooped up without access to accurate information or any hope for a return to something that feels normal, and you have met all your creative goals already, have even taken to googling "bucket list" just to see what other people hope to someday accomplish, although you remain uninspired.

Why is six afraid of seven? You name it. That cough, Trump supporter, climate change, gun violence, bad breath, weird around his daughter. Who isn't afraid of seven right now? Not like six is much better. Coronavirus denialist.

There are a few easy ways to manage boredom. One tried-and-true method is to develop rituals that divide your day into manageable parcels of time. (You may find that you do this outside of captivity, too, for example by going into the office.) Ideally these rituals will aid you in both mind and body—exercise, say, as opposed to smoking—but really the name of the game is whatever it takes to get through the day. If cutting calms you best right now, just make sure to disinfect your blades.

Why did the chicken cross the road? Boredom, duh. Who wouldn't cross a road right now if they could? I would kill to cross a fucking road.

If you wake in the morning to a sixteen-hour stretch of nothingness, try meditating for twenty minutes, three times per day. Then you will only have fifteen hours without structure, some of which will be taken up by dreading meditation. Skin-care rituals may also be worth cultivating. Endless hours can be spent staring into the mirror pretending that various balms and ointments have barely perceptible effects. Cardio is recommended by numerous medical professionals and personal trainers, although it can also be a little boring. Baking, knitting, video games: there are many activities. Washing dishes! Anything to which your immediate gut reaction is "WASTE OF TIME." That shit is your BFF rn.

Yo mama is so lying in a hospital right now, hooked up to a respirator, dying alone. You won't be able to attend the funeral.

You may occasionally ask yourself, "Aren't I just killing time here? And since I don't know how much longer I'll be in captivity, might it not be weird to waste what could be an endless number of days, in fact what could be all my remaining time on Earth or, if I am very young, make up my entire existence?" It is good to ask questions that consider the root of human existence. However, you may soon realize that the basic purpose of asking such questions is to raise them in a debate forum with other humans in the back corner of a local drinking establishment, and as such, these questions do little at this moment to serve you. Consider them all you like. You may even develop strong feelings regarding various potential answers. But unless questions offer improvement to your existence within an immediate time frame—say, four hours—you may find that the answers do not matter.

What's black and white and read all over? No one has any idea anymore. Is there even such a thing?

What you probably miss most is the surprising nature of people doing things that you yourself would not think of or care to do. Perhaps something so simple as laugh at a joke, or more complex, like bake a cake for your birthday. Maybe it's a coworker tripping you, perhaps on purpose. Do you miss that? That tiny recognition that the presence of other people can influence your life in profound ways, good or bad? Human contact of any kind? The idea that someone would care so much about where you are going and why you are going there that they wish to stop you in your tracks but refrain from doing you any permanent bodily damage?

Knock, knock. Who's there. Literally anyone. Please do not touch the door handle, sir. You can leave the delivery on the front stoop, and I will collect it in three days.

Try wrapping yourself in cling wrap. If it works for fifties housewives, it will probably work for you! Or text yourself to ask, "Is your refrigerator running?" and when you reply that it is, suggest to yourself that you better go catch it! Poke a tiny hole in an egg and let the insides drip out, and then replace the empty shell in your egg carton. When you later crack it open and discover nothing inside, you will be delighted! And possibly annoyed with yourself. But the good news is that you will now have to spend a day trying to find more eggs. Activities!

A bear and a rabbit are in the woods. The rabbit says to the bear, "What's that smell?" and the bear goes, "Smell? I don't . . . oh shit, feel my forehead. Do I have a fever?"

If you have a spray attachment for your kitchen sink, affix a rubber band tightly around the handle before you go to sleep at night. When you wake up in the morning, you will be delighted and surprised to suddenly be covered in cold water! Maybe not delighted. Also, this won't work if you are literally glued head to toe to your bed, or stuck in the bottom of a well. In the well, you may be able to emulate the experience by standing in the rain, or splashing a bit from the standing pool of water while thinking really hard about something else. Try not to drink any! It would not be smart to catch typhoid fever if you are already afflicted with the ailment of being stuck in a well.

Take my wife. She'll go out to the grocery store, no mask, start screaming at the cashiers, "This is America! This is America!" Take my wife—please! I can't take her anymore myself. Thousands of people are dying every day!

In conclusion, there may never be a conclusion. You may be in captivity for months, or years, or intermittently throughout the next decade! No one knows. Worse: it might never be funny.

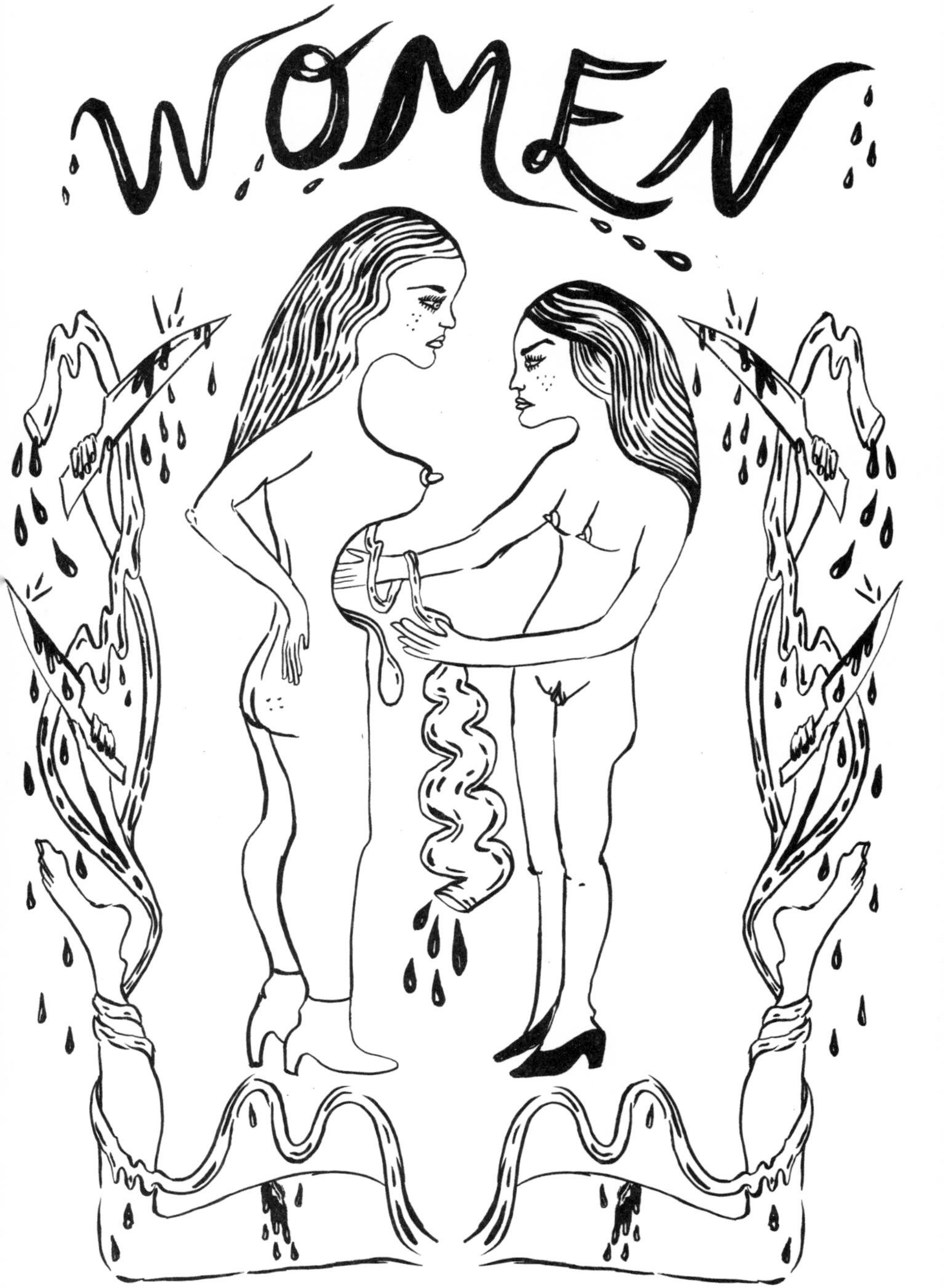
WOMEN

ARGUABLY, LUCKY MCKEE'S *The Woman*—heralded in promotional materials as the "most controversial film" of its release year, 2011—is nothing more than a close study of justifiable misogyny. Not the low-level, no-girls-allowed stuff we can still stumble across on occasion these days, but a thorough hatred of the insufficiently masculine as ideology, as spirituality. A sustained rejection of femininity, manifested in a violence so wretched and grotesque it becomes all-consuming, self-explanatory, and deeply righteous. It leaks from on-screen characters and encompasses the theater, the living room. Viewers of McKee's film are placed, for a time, in the uncanny position of acquiescence to a religion they may not believe in. It is uncomfortable. For although I live in a world that demands my destruction in a myriad of ways every day and I have thus learned to follow the logic of misogyny, I have no desire to *feel* it.

McKee's film lays its groundwork carefully. A five-minute opening sequence follows a feral woman through the woods. She is nurturing and careful, but also blood-sucking and unkempt, so definitely wild. A jump cut to Peggy, the teenage daughter of a happy-enough-seeming family at a backyard barbecue—isolated and disconsolate—establishes this film as one about *gender issues*. Heavy-handed, but not unclever, McKee then ticks off a list of familial dysfunctions as the rest of the clan parades across the screen. Peggy's brother, Brian, watches with glazed eyes as his youngest sister, Darlin', gets roughed up by neighborhood boys. Their mother, Belle (played by an unusually unhinged Angela Bettis), acts deflective and abused around her husband, even in public, even at a party. Upon repeated viewings, it's clear we are witnessing emotionally and sexually abused family members reenact their domestic roles for neighborhood innocents, but you don't so much notice this on first viewing.

And that husband, Chris Cleek (Sean Bridgers). There is nothing remarkable about him. He is brash and aggravating, and believes his jokes to be very funny. You have met him several times at barbecues yourself. He is a lawyer, and he likes to hunt. When he goes off into the woods some time later, he finds the Woman there, in the wild, through the sight of his rifle. A deep bass line kicks in, the scene goes slo-mo, and we are suddenly in a rock video. She emerges from the water and arches her back, sexually, for him, as she redresses herself. He wants her, and not just to fuck. He wants to own her: a possession, a catch, a prize.

So he takes her. Chains her up in the cellar, and eventually introduces her to the family. Not as a person, but as his thing, to wash and feed and use at will. Of course for sex—she's not a person in his mind, but a masturbation aid. She isn't human, she's a wild woman, but also just a woman. The metaphors fall away quickly, thin veils that, until this moment, have kept Chris Cleek and by extension every other self-important lawyer/hunter/father you've ever met at a backyard family barbecue from going on a rape-and-murder rampage. The veils are labeled—society, respect, family, love—and when the last one falls away, we have only the patriarch, finally unhinged but honest, ranting against womanhood as he pummels every female within spitting distance to the ground.

In the last twenty minutes of the film, there are no more metaphors, only raw and pure misogyny explored to its fullest, without restraint. It is messy and sticky, like an underserved man's well-earned orgasm. Belle, too late, speaks up. This is not tolerated. A meddling lesbian teacher, interfering, accidently unearths a family secret. She is punished. Peggy balks. She is beaten. Brian, revealed to be the psychopath and rapist he has been trained to be throughout his entire life, is rewarded. Finally, the men—having imposed total dominion over the women—set to tearing one another apart. And then the tables are turned, sort of, although maybe put back where they belong?

We'll return to those, the discomfiting final moments of the film, and pause to answer the question surely forming in your mind: How is this not the most offensive and depraved hate speech ever dressed up as entertainment and put on public display in the history of man? The studio's marketing team would like you to believe that it is, although this is mere marketing. This film is not exclusively a performance *of* misogyny; it posits that misogyny might emanate, also, from women. It therefore imagines an abiding detestation of femininity as something over which women may have control, even agency. *The Woman* degenders the misogynist, allowing misogyny a pervasiveness and a logic that very closely mirrors reality. Believe it or not, that misogyny might exist in all of us is, actually, quite a hopeful notion.

♠ ♠ ♠

Let's consider this about misogyny: if we want to lay all the blame for all the problems of the world at the feet of men—aka the patriarchy—we certainly may. Plenty of people do, and they make their arguments quite well, whether dusty academics or eleven-year-old girls on TikTok. There exists plenty of evidence to back up such claims. The adoration of the masculine as protector must also decry the feminine in all nonsubmissive forms, and who better to advance such a ridiculous notion than men?

Unfortunately, "because men" doesn't provide a terribly satisfactory answer to the question of how a deep, anti-feminine undercurrent came to run through all of culture and society, providing a humming ethos for our very socioeconomic structure and daily interactions. To hold as true that misogyny is inescapable but emanates exclusively from cis men, we must also believe one of two things: (1) that women and nonbinary people, who truly do exist in every corner of society, even if we cannot see them or do not acknowledge them, in point of fact do have no power, or (2) that women and nonbinary people are party to the same flawed thinking as anyone else, as cis men, as the patriarchy, and therefore tend to use what power they do have toward disastrous ends, at least where gender equality may be concerned. The first construct strips women of agency—itself a misogynist act—while the second degenders misogyny and makes women complicit in it, blaming them, in part, for their own oppression. Yet it also offers a modicum of control over an otherwise external, and often overwhelming, force.

These strokes are overly broad and the gender binary they rely on easily disprovable, but the question I'm getting at is this: Would we rather our cultural products *perform* misogyny, or hold folks accountable for it? We could push this question further, for even an abiding belief in the gender binary is an act of violence against those who do not fall neatly into it: Would we rather *perform* transmisogyny or hold folks accountable for it?[1]

Most of us familiar with the term, in hoping to ultimately eliminate the need for it, would likely prefer a notion of misogyny that held folks accountable for gender-based violence in all forms. For filmmakers, however, the question is not always so simple. Consider, for example, Lars von Trier's *Antichrist*. "Accusations of misogyny are routine in discussions of Mr. von Trier's films," the *New York Times* summarized in a 2014 review of *Nymphomaniac*, following a tally of the harsh brutalities his leads are forced to endure throughout his oeuvre.[2] (Rape by gang of sailors, rape by entire town, genital mutilation, and murder are such standard von Trier fodder that many were disappointed that 2011's *Melancholia* merely ended with the world melting. Spoiler alert!)

The *Times*, however, decreed von Trier *not* a misogynist, based on ample evidence the director himself has supplied, proving he believes women to be capable of performing under the most extreme circumstances in his films, upholding their narratives in the entirety in almost every single case. Indeed, the evidence for von Trier's nonmisogyny grows, for he himself found his original draft of *Antichrist* to be *not misogynist enough*, so he hired "misogyny expert" Heidi Laura, *a woman*, to deepen the hatred of femininity that undergirds the film.

For the film performers von Trier works with, the answer to the question I pose above is easy: they would rather perform misogyny—that is, perform the experience of it. They do so commendably. It is not in their job descriptions to hold anyone accountable to anything, and performing actual misogyny has got to be a far cry more interesting than mildly reflecting it as the girlfriend or mother of a protagonist, who may not even have a name, much less a battle scar. The hope of such actors, expressed in countless interviews and public statements, is to perform something well enough that indictment will follow—although by others, and later.

For von Trier the question is more complicated: He wants to put on a performance of misogyny, but he wants to do it deliberately. So well, in fact, that he will find the folks who know the most about its effects and pay them to provide pointers on the stuff, even if they are women, because there are many, many things that they are better at than men. (Suffering, apparently, is another skill he evidently believes women hold unique talent in.) His is a thoughtful performance of misogyny, and I submit that we are intended to believe that its aim is to hold others accountable for unchecked, undeliberate, unthoughtful misogyny elsewhere.

Yet the women in von Trier's films tend to accept devastation, and that's worth considering too: even Justine, Kirsten Dunst's lead in *Melancholia*, submits to the world-ending scenario despite her otherwise narcissistic behavior, making no effort to shift the course of nature toward something more befitting her own interests, which otherwise dominate the plotline of the film. Von Trier may be orchestrating a performance of misogyny with a considered delivery and purposeful intent, but his leading ladies hardly bother kicking against the pricks. The world they collectively envision in his films either allows for a great deal of unchecked feminine disapproval, or it will destroy itself and they will submit to it. Von Trier's misogyny may be intentionally constructed, in other words, but without agency, his women characters are still left to its whims. They are not hopeful films.

Lucky McKee, arguably a lesser artist with a much tinier vision—certainly a genre filmmaker—takes a far more expansive view. His horrific universe is filled with horrible people committing horrible acts, too, although another possibility can be detected in his films: a future in which misogyny may be eradicated. What might it take to build that world? At the end of *The Woman*, we begin to have a sense.

▲ ▲ ▲

"We belong to the gender of fear, of humiliation, to the alien gender," French theorist and filmmaker Virginie Despentes writes in *King Kong Theory*, whereas men simply belong: in the world, together. "This exclusion of our bodies is the foundation on which masculinity is built. . . . A pact based on our inferiority."[3] It is observation, but also prescription. By acknowledging the site of misogyny—in women's own fear, humiliation, and alienness—she begins to perceive her own complicity in it.

Despentes offers a corrective. She suggests eliminating that wellspring of gendered fear, humiliation, and alienness with a display of power. Describing her own violent rape after hitchhiking to a concert, she opines the boredom that might otherwise have overcome her. Going out into a violent hypermasculine world, she says, was "worth putting yourself in danger for. Nothing could be worse than being holed up in my bedroom, cut off from life, when there was so much happening out there."[4] She will not apologize for brazenness, or dwell in her naivete. Instead she opts to acknowledge the danger by walking toward it. By experiencing it. And by moving on.

During her own rape, she had a knife that she did not use. She writes eloquently of the long history of feminine indoctrination into nonviolence, a long-standing strategy that keeps women from defending themselves. "But," she writes, "when the day comes that men are afraid of having their dicks hacked off with a box cutter if they force themselves on a woman, they'll learn pretty quickly to control their 'manly' urges."[5]

This strategy of indoctrination is one she terms political, but effective. Even when her own bodily integrity was at stake, then violated, she felt herself pushed—by fear—to honor the physical sanctity of her rapist. Despentes detects, in other words, her own misogyny. She was complacent to rape, allowed it to take place at the site of her own body, let herself become evidence of it, proof that misogyny lived within her. Not a condition she was all that amenable to, in the end: she writes that she would have preferred to carve it from the necks of her attackers—cutting it symbolically out of herself—than to live with it inside her.

But for her indoctrination into the political strategy that is rape, perhaps Despentes would have defended herself with an equal violence. Certainly, however, she would have taken less time to comprehend her rape as rape, to name it, to speak about it at all. She writes that it took years.

Mine did too. Less violent, far more social—and therefore more difficult to identify, at first. But it did help spark the realization that as an editor, I tended to discredit submissions from women writers. Soon my own disregard for feminized labor—care work like nursing and early childhood education—started to become clear to me. I grew to understand that the sense I grew up with, that other young women were competition instead of allies, was instilled in me from elsewhere, that other young women were going through many of the same things I was, and sometimes wanted to share burdens and experiences. I began to see that the patriarchy wasn't keeping women down: I was. Learning to hate other women had taken time too. My complacency to misogyny was honed over years of watching good, kind, well-meaning friends comply to the gender-based oppression on display in others, and embodying it themselves. My own rape should probably have been years earlier, in fact, as I was trained by a violent, racist, overbearing, alcoholic father to comply to his every whim from birth, rewarded every time I did by the authority figures in my life. Yet by the time it happened (at a party, there was drinking, everyone was pushing boundaries, verbal consent impossible in a foreign country where language skills are shaky), it felt so thoroughly natural that it took me a decade to notice a violation had occurred. By the time I named it rape, it was already far in the past. By accepting it, unnamed, for so many years, I know that I have the capacity to overlook it if it happens again right in front of me. It is possible that I will let it happen to someone else. Perhaps I already have.

What I know, therefore, is that the fear, humiliation, and alienness Despentes points to—they need to be stamped out. In myself and in others. Unlike Despentes, if I went back and slit the throats of everyone directly complicit in my rape, the bodies left open and bleeding would not only be those of men. That, in fact, is part of why it took so long for me to identify my experience as rape: because I did not fully understand how capable of misogyny women can be. I thought my feminine friends by definition could not stand by and watch my bodily integrity be violated. Now I remember a time that they did.

If I could borrow Despentes's box cutter and slash the misogyny from my favorite female friends, I certainly would. The submissive, accepting reaction of women to a dominant, violent culture, the way that they—we—have conformed to and upheld a dynamic that has stripped women of agency and which they—we—have accepted without adjustment—if I could find it in their bodies I would carve it out. If I could locate it in myself I would remove it and watch it die.

▲ ▲ ▲

Film depictions of rape are diverse and telling. Take the classic rape-revenge fantasy *I Spit on Your Grave*. Originally released under the superior title *Day of the Woman*, Meir Zarchi's 1978 film is brilliant, horror or no, rape-revenge fantasy or no. Although replete with unexamined class problems—the idle rich win out over the struggling poor in the end—there are few more accurate depictions of American culture than this little gem.

What distressed American viewing audiences (and why you may never have heard of it) is that the film takes Despentes's pronouncement—that rape may be controllable if women learn to defend themselves with violence—seriously. And because it does, both the critical reception and the viewership of the film have been curtailed. The lesson to be learned here is how deeply abiding misogyny is, and how intrinsic to capitalism.

The film follows an urban transplant, writer Jennifer Hills, during her summer sojourn in the country by the lake. Her tranquility is broken, repeatedly, by four young men from town, and she grows agitated. Eventually, they nab her, bring her to a remote area of the forest, and rape her brutally and repeatedly. When they finally leave, we witness her struggle to stand and then slowly return home; there they await her and, again, attack. Three of the young men leave after convincing a fourth, who has some form of intellectual impairment, to kill her. He cannot, but later claims that he did. Her recovery takes weeks, and when she reemerges, the group of rapists turn on one another in fury that she survived. United they may have been a threat, but once divided, she seduces each handily. Coitus interruptus: she then kills each attacker brutally. It is remorseless and ever-so-slightly thrilling.

Jennifer does this impassively, played by a sensibly stoic Camille Keaton, Buster's granddaughter. That she married Zarchi before the film found distribution undercuts the force of the narrative a bit: on-screen she is a serenely composed, self-aware, independent woman, both before and then a while after the rape. Her stage presence is commanding: it alone is worth audiencefuls of appreciation. Yet can a woman be depicted as remorseless without a supportive, off-screen husband?

Critics didn't care, and panned it out of hand (inspiring a cult following, of course). Roger Ebert gave it zero stars and called it a "vile bag of garbage. . . . Sick, reprehensible and contemptible," getting the thrust of the film dead wrong overall but sprinkling in a muted, off-key cheer for "feminist solidarity."[6] (Barf.) He never let it go. Years later, in an *Oprah Winfrey Show* appearance with Gene Siskel, the two laugh heartily when an audience member asks Ebert to name the worst film he's ever seen. The longtime colleagues both know the answer: *I Spit on Your Grave*. *Tasteless*, *irresponsible*, and *disturbing* are common insults hurled at the film by critics, and certain characters receive unfair portions of blame: namely the "retarded" rapist Ebert points to and the "sick," "sadistic," "degraded" female protagonist described by the film's many dismissive critics. Britain used the film to push for tighter control over film standards—censorship. Without the cult following the critical animosity inspired—and the simultaneous rise of the videocassette-rental industry—the film would have been effectively buried.

Carol J. Clover attempted to set the record straight in her 1992 book *Men, Women, and Chain Saws*. Providing an overview of the film's negative critical reception, she qualifies its inclusion in her tome on gender and horror by restating the purpose of her book: "to offer an account not just of the most but also the least presentable of horror," nearly apologizing for the nod to the existence of the offensive garbage that is *I Spit on Your Grave*.[7] She says that she does not "fully share" the negative views of the film—noting one interviewee's suggestion that it be made compulsory viewing on high school campuses—and identifies the film as not as shocking and less valueless than critics charged. She further suggests that it fails primarily because it never adopted a masculinist viewpoint, in which gang rape would be let off the hook as acceptable, and makes excellent points about individual culpability for violent actions—each rapist blames the others, at some point, or blames the victim, which begins to raise larger questions about how rape occurs. Yet whatever social value she may find in the film, Clover ultimately condemns it as artless.

It's not true—long, ponderous scenes of tranquility and solitude effectively underscore the plotline of the film, which lend it quite an arty sense indeed—but more interesting is Clover's point about the gendered POV of the film. If it is true that Zarchi's film failed to adopt a masculinist viewpoint, and that this caused meltdowns in both the reviews section of the newspaper and at the box office, we can surmise quite a bit about how allegiant we expect culture to be to the logic of rape and misogyny.

Strongly allegiant, it's safe to say. Let's take the subgenre of horror the film sits in as a first example. From a certain perspective, contextualizing a film as rape-revenge fantasy is a problem in itself. We do not have burglary-revenge-fantasy films, although plenty of movies begin with a thieved item and continue under a plot dictated by its reacquisition. Movies in which kidnappers or terrorists are hunted down are not characterized as kidnapping- or terrorism-revenge fantasies. Kidnapping and terrorism are too correctly situated already as legitimate crimes to need to justify them as revenge worthy. Too, films in which rapes of women occur in the first place are not termed woman-revenge-fantasy flicks. In fact, sometimes they are just fantasy, if they are distinguished in any way at all. Rape, in fact, is the standard. In horror, in film, and in culture. Only retaliation against it is marked and unusual.

This is not to say that rape is inevitable, or common, or necessary: only that we do not condemn it thoroughly whenever it occurs. I didn't, when it happened to me.

Untold numbers of women don't, either, some perhaps operating under confusion about what does and does not constitute rape. Such confusion is more common in some circles than others—as Missouri Congressional Representative Todd Akin's 2012 claims of the impossibility of pregnancy in the case of "legitimate" rape indicate, as well as, a decade later, the sheer disbelief among GOP pundits that a ten-year-old may have been subject to a rape that would have necessitated a newly criminalized abortion in her home state in 2022. Cultural confusion allows for a legal one. As Despentes writes, "When it comes to rape, you have to keep on proving you weren't up for it."[8] In *I Spit on Your Grave*, Jennifer doesn't bother proving anything to anyone. She simply extracts revenge.

I Spit on Your Grave allows for a cultural imaginary in which the domain of women is violence, both serene and justified, as Despentes suggests it should be. But culture has a way of enforcing adherence to norms, even if tiny pockets of resistance can be found; few know this as well as Despentes, who has also made films that were considered rape-revenge fantasies and were censored. Her theory therefore proves out—that "rape is a clear-cut political stratagem: the skeletal frame of capitalism."[9]

In the end, capitalism marked *I Spit on Your Grave*. The film was problematized by critics like Ebert, who labeled it a deviation from the standard and acceptable depiction of gender politics. (What damning praise, this "feminist solidarity"!) Then the film was censored, for those same reasons. Distribution was limited, screenings short when held at all. The domino effect continued. Streaming platforms, at first, didn't offer it; now it's housed on free sites, relegated to the realm of mindless, valueless gore. The film developed a small cult audience upon release made possible by newly emerging specialty video-rental stores and still enjoys one today: perhaps the best capitalism can do for feminine subjects, in the end.

For fans of narrative diversity, as well as those who would prefer the eradication of misogyny, this presents a real problem. The fatal flaw of *I Spit on Your Grave*, a truly great film, is that it fails to privilege a masculinist worldview. This kept it from wider distribution, critical acclaim, and audiences of all but the most dedicated genre enthusiasts. Could *I Spit on Your Grave* function as a social imaginary, allowing a possible future in which more men refrain from sexual assault out of fear of getting their dicks cut off in bathtubs? We simply don't know, in this political economy: people would have to see it first.

▲ ▲ ▲

So we do not have *Day of the Woman* to look to, but we do have *The Woman*. The 2011 film somehow escapes the problematic rape-revenge framing—because Chris Cleek carries the bulk of the narrative? Because there's so much more rape in it than revenge?—but otherwise is set against this same sordid history. My theory is that what popular success McKee's film has seen is due to its overt contention that women deserve the oppression they get. Most of the run time of the film, in fact, is obsessively devoted to its masculinist viewpoint—the one so lacking in *I Spit on Your Grave*.

In McKee's tale, every female character eventually cannibalizes, consuming herself or others due to starvation, mistreatment, or a fear that is misunderstood to be love. You can read this as a metaphor if you like, but some of these women straight-up eat people. It is a cultural mandate, yes: in this world dominated by a hateful lawyer and his shitty rapist asshole serial killer son, the only means of feminine survival is to sacrifice your body or that of the nearest replacement female. You might starve if you do not consume the flesh of another. Women on-screen hold equal responsibility to men on-screen for the oppression of women, no question. (One of the smart turns of the film is that certain bizarre leaps in plot are blamed on a female character's unrelated medical condition, anophthalmia, the absence of one or both eyes. She is unable to see. Women in *The Woman* are horrible, we can surmise by extension, because they *are incapable of perceiving the world.*)

Then McKee's film veers off course. Until then a stunning metaphor for present-day sexual politics, the narrative falters in its resolution. In the final moments of the film, the feminine returns to nature and nurture, and the masculine is left to rule society and culture: a false dichotomy based on a misguided assertion that gender is biological and cultural politics rooted therein. We will not be offered a view of a world in which women make violence their permanent domain within an existing culture; McKee has women stepping back from society entirely, allowing it to remain the dominion of men.

A truly radical narrative might have destroyed this false dichotomy, already breached, or supplanted each with each: What would a society look like if women simply protected themselves in the world into which they are born? Then again, a truly radical film would have featured a soundtrack and production by people who are not men, thus creating an economic infrastructure to support feminine cast and crew (as, somewhat awkwardly, von Trier occasionally does). A visionary filmmaker might even have followed through on Despentes's suggestion that men can learn to refrain from rape and women can learn to embrace the violence of self-protection, and given us a glimpse of what that might look like. It's probably horrifying.

The Woman isn't, therefore, a radical feminist film. But by siting misogyny in women, it offers a glimpse of a future in which it can be controlled and from which it can be eradicated.

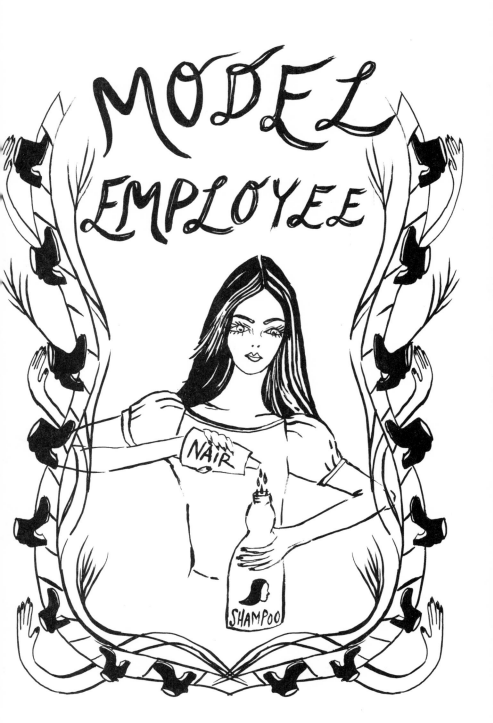

"MY MOM WAS A model, and I was expected to follow in her footsteps," Sarah Meier tells me over Skype from her home in Manila. At fourteen she did, living the NYC top-model lifestyle for twelve years before moving back home to work on a radio show and as an MTV VJ. She was even set to host *Philippines' Next Top Model* before the show was canceled, when she took a gig editing the country's premier fashion magazine, *Metro*. I feel compelled to mention that she's got big green eyes; long, straight hair; and glowing, flawless skin. She's beautiful. It is, after all, an important part of her job.

What I'm impressed by, however, is Meier's thoughtfulness. She spent over a decade attending up to ten castings per day, each filled with panels of critics offering professional and often conflicting opinions about her physical flaws. It started to wear, she explains. After a few years, she says she felt a creeping sense of self-doubt. It afflicted others too.

"Really, really, really nice girls turned into horrible creatures," she says. She's referring to her endless string of model roommates. The agencies that administer model contracts also arrange for housing, but the expenses come out of employee paychecks, a standard fashion-industry variation on the sharecroppers' company store. The day a new roomie moved in was always great, Meier recalls. But, she adds, "Three months down the road, they're putting Nair in each other's shampoo bottles."

Reality may be crueler than reality television, but the real-life travails of models don't necessarily arise out of professional rivalry. "You could be looking at a blond-haired, blue-eyed girl, and you're not in competition with her at all"—Meier has light-brown skin and dark-brown hair—"we're not going to be up for the same jobs, ever. We're not even sent to the same castings. But the way in which we view each other is competition. Like, 'Do you have a better body?' 'How can you get away with eating that when I'm here suffering?' The animosity begins to build. Not just animosity for other models. It becomes animosity for anybody that's happy. Anybody that's living a normal life."

Close students of class politics will recognize Meier's cutting flourish as a textbook description of proletarian alienation. Except, of course, few of us are inclined to think of models as workers. To judge by their portfolios, models spend an inordinate amount of time at swanky cocktail soirees, cavorting on Caribbean beaches, or drunkenly weaving down urban thoroughfares, laughing at passersby with their high-heeled shoes in their hands. Yet even models like Meier, at the top of the modeling food chain in New York, can find the stylized mimicry of the good life they perform for the camera an intolerable, degrading grind. And with vicious campaigns of interpersonal one-upmanship as virtual conditions of employment, a spectator might consider looking beyond the images of la dolce vita studiously crafted by the industry to ponder just what kind of self is being assembled as an object of choice for ornamentation and adornment.

In other words, toxicity is inherent to the modeling caste: doled out to all comers, no minor glitch in an otherwise efficient system but a condition of the job. It is, in short, a labor issue.

♦ ♦ ♦

The charge that models have a rough go of it, however, has not yet caught the popular imagination. After all, the posh surface of the industry gleams with overclass self-indulgence. Even the breed of feminist politically awakened by a T-shirt slogan can tick off the profession's glaring ideological sins: its misogynist conflation of Woman, always, with salable object; its role in lionizing impossible-to-maintain beauty standards; and its casual enactment of reflexive female consent in the realm of sexual power—the complex of predatory prerogatives we've come to name rape culture. As a result, labor activists and feminists alike suffer an understandable exasperation when confronting otherwise-prosaic labor concerns. Fighting for fair wages or adequate child labor protections in an industry so steeped in—foundational to—the iconography of male privilege can seem like petitioning the Koch brothers to join Code Pink.

Then comes a sneaking suspicion that most models haven't spent enough time in the real world to fully comprehend that unjust treatment may not be heaped upon them because of their job, but because of their gender. A cognitive dissonance arises when a seemingly pampered sector of the leisure class stumbles upon a millennia-old pattern of gender oppression as though its members were the first group to encounter it. Why should I care about pay equity in the modeling industry, in other words, when I suffer it daily as a journalist and college professor?

Modeling is, by any reasonable measure of working-class drudgery, a decidedly elite career. Even insiders, pointing out unfair labor practices, describe an "exclusive . . . hyper-wealthy country club—like industry" and complain that agencies take too high a percentage of presumably lavish salaries.[1]

Indeed, Meier prefers to characterize her taste of the lush life in positive terms. "I know what a really expensive car feels like to sit in. I know what it smells like," she tells me. "I've tasted some really incredible food and seen some really beautiful places in the world." But country clubs and expensive cars come staffed, a nuance some may overlook. Former cover girl Jennifer Sky, in a call for actors' union SAG-AFTRA to grant models entry, casually mentioned that in her model apartment, "We didn't pick up after ourselves or clean the floor."[2] It's hard to work up much in the way of labor solidarity for people who seem to feel they are the deserved beneficiaries of labor but aren't, you know, *laborers*.

As the rallying cry for models to organize has gained volume in recent years, the cause of solidarity with other labor sectors has lagged. What models do is sell, not construct or argue or plan, and any effort to stir them into militancy inevitably ends up navigating the narrow catwalk between cause marketing and genuine labor organizing. Visiting the website for the advocacy group Model Alliance in 2015, for example, opened a pop-up ad for a sexy-lady calendar that temporarily blocked you from reading a draft of the Models' Bill of Rights.[3] The calendar "features twelve models who the Alliance feels represent female empowerment and diversity in the American modeling industry," according to the site.[4] Sure enough, the sexualized pouts of twelve women smizing through a variety of skin tones adorn the months of the year. The draft bill of rights, on the other hand, proposed concrete measures to end wage theft, ensure fiscal oversight of agencies, and minimize child labor—decidedly unsexy fare, especially when set against the calendar's high-gloss array of seductive poses. The master's tools may not dismantle the master's house, but check out how great they look in action!

Yet when you peer beyond the pouts and cognitive dissonance, you gradually come to realize that the struggles facing the women paid to act out patriarchal notions of beauty, glamour, and worldliness are not so different from those that assail the figures with whom we've long associated the intersection of fashion and politics: underpaid and overworked garment-factory employees. Neither, for that matter, are models' demands much different from those we hear from any other woman involved in the global garment trade, at any phase of production or distribution.

⬥ ⬥ ⬥

My first peek inside a garment factory, in Cambodia in 2009, was a quick one. People who don't work there are not usually allowed in, and certainly journalists are denied entry out of hand, so I lied to the guard in Khmer and faked a heedlessness common to Americans traveling in Southeast Asia. I breezed through the entryway, gaily commenting on the rumbling in my stomach as I headed toward a crowd of young women at a picnic table. The guard caught me after two steps. "It is not a restaurant," he told me in gruff Cambodian syllables. "You must leave."

He glanced at his weapon—an AK-47, the ubiquity of the guns a holdover from the Khmer Rouge era—so I exited the factory gates and joined a crew of mostly young women in the back of another Pol Pot holdover, a decommissioned Chinese military vehicle. My translator joined me to help ask them about their jobs. At first they didn't respond, only shared with me their meager lunch. There is no freedom of press in Cambodia, and workers are explicitly warned not to speak to reporters. My translator told them not to worry, that I was just a tourist who likes clothes. This characterization of me as a guileless fashion fan cheered them, and they agreed, finally, to answer questions.

They were, in all senses, model employees: adorable, pleasant, and happy in their jobs. This last strained my credulity, as it was a blisteringly hot day—they all are, inside the factories—and the five young women and single young man in the back of the truck didn't have enough food, but couldn't afford more. In 2009 the monthly minimum wage was only $50. (In 2023 this will go up to $200 per month, but the cost of living is rising, too, and unions are demanding a minimum hike to $206.[5]) Statistically, we'd need another three and a half women to jam themselves in the back of the tiny truck to represent the current gender ratio of the Cambodian factory workforce, but there simply wasn't room.

Some in this group packed jeans to ship to China and North America, although it's rare for workers to know where wares end up. Under global Fordism, most grasp only what passes through their field of vision, and the fashion industry is notoriously decentralized. Nearly all that's required to establish a garment's provenance under international trade regulations is the momentary labor of sewing in a "Made In" label—the primary means by which globalization can be tracked by consumers.

Still, the destination of most Southeast Asian–made garments is predictable: At the time, 70 percent of all apparel produced in Cambodia was imported to the United States. Nowadays, around 45 percent goes to the EU and around 30 percent to the US, although production has increased during this time too.[6] While Asian countries, particularly China, lead denim exports, the US still drives consumption of those, too, accounting for around 40 percent of jeans purchased worldwide. Unlike most apparel, these jeans are made in a single factory: the sole man in the lunch bunch was a cutter from the very front of the line, an unusual find in a gathering of workers who pack final garments for shipping.

Yet his placement at the earliest stage of production didn't offer a substantial difference in vantage point on the group's complaints of labor abuses, many of which were reminiscent of the early days of the Industrial Revolution. The International Labour Organization (ILO)–backed monitoring agent Better Factories Cambodia (BFC) regularly documents the extent to which Asian garment work remains impervious to basic labor and safety regulations. During the 2008 inspections, monitors discovered that some factories weren't meeting minimum wage pay standards, particularly for casual workers, whose ranks only increased after the global economic recession later that same year.[7] Legally required maternity leave pay was granted to only three-quarters of the workers who requested it; only two-thirds of workers requesting sick pay received it. And even these discouraging numbers don't track the vast group of workers who have not been informed of their rights to demand them. Half the companies in the ILO survey failed to meet basic health and safety requirements, and 92 percent were found to illegally mandate overtime work. Wage theft was frequent, commonly carried out through management flacks, who omitted or mischaracterized pay stub translations to employees who were unable to read. Health facilities, mandatory under Cambodian law, remained understaffed, when they were available at all.

More recent, reliable reports are hard to track down. In 2012 questions about the effectiveness of BFC's close ties to the government and the garment industry were raised at the same time that the Better Factories program was replicated in other nations; current inspection reports are not available on the Better Factories website, replaced by less detailed reports on factory compliance with national COVID-19 guidelines. Yet there's little cause to hope that factories have suddenly improved working conditions, drastically or at all: the Clean Clothes Campaign, working with Cambodian trade unions, estimated that the nearly eight hundred thousand workers in the country's garment industry lost a total $393 million to wage theft, outstanding wages, and withheld severance pay during the first year of the pandemic.

When I asked the Cambodian workers in that truck about their prospects in the industry, it became clear how differently women and men view garment work as a career. I wanted to know if the women hoped to advance in the factory in the future, for example, but they only smiled. My translator prodded them with greater eloquence, but this had no effect. Finally, I asked outright, "Would you like to be managers?"

The women broke into raucous laughter. "Oh, they would like," my translator explained through their giggled uproar. "But no time." Time to study accounting, earn a high school degree, attend college, he continued, which would also take money. Most of their funds—only fifty-five dollars per month, keep in mind—were sent back home to support family farms. That's why young people in Cambodia get sent to the city to work in the first place. Approximately 20 percent of the country's nearly seventeen million residents survive on the incomes of eight hundred thousand workers in today's garment trade. The family tradition of shipping daughters off to work leaves Cambodia's already weak bureaucratic state scrambling to document the ever-widening epidemic of underage labor. Official documents are easy to fake and not always required, and a young person's genuine interest in helping the family may mean she's willing to lie about her age, even if she knows her real birth date, which several generations of Cambodians do not. So while underage workers throng the garment factories, reliable statistics on the problem of child labor are almost impossible to collect. Women at the time face other barriers to advancement too: only 4 percent of the garment factory managers in the country are women, most of whom are owners' relatives.[8] For these young women to advance in the factories, in other words, they would have to have been born into the business.

The young man stayed silent as his feminine coworkers described their fates. He knew that he would probably make manager if he wanted to, or get another job if he didn't. His colleagues also lacked the simple sovereignty over their own persons that he was more likely to be able

to take for granted. A 2020 report from Better Factories Cambodia found that between 40 and 60 percent of
women workers reported experiencing sexual harassment
in the workplace, and 10 percent of men.[9]

My hosts' twenty-minute lunch break ended quickly,
and they waved goodbye. In a few hours, three of the
youngest would walk home together after work, to the
cramped factory housing unit they shared with three other
young women to save money, and make a meager dinner.
After that, they'd fall asleep right away because it would
be late, and because they would have to get up early the
next day and do it all over again.

▲ ▲ ▲

We recognize labor and human rights violations when
they occur on the production end of global fashion, but
any close look at the display sector will reveal a distressing litany of similarities—beginning with the tendencies
of garment factories and modeling agencies alike to prey
on young women. (A feature they share with the marketing divisions that stoke demand for the products of both
industries.)

"It's a brutal world," Meier says, recalling her entry into
the display-side workforce. "They do want you to come
in at the age of thirteen, fourteen, hoping that you'll hit
your prime at seventeen." A 2012 Model Alliance report,
not yet repeated, found that more than half the models
surveyed had started between thirteen and sixteen;
another 1 percent had started earlier. More than half of
those underage were never or were rarely accompanied
by a legal guardian to castings or jobs. (The Model Alliance

sample size was small—85 completed surveys, from the 241 who received the form—but so is the modeling world. The US Bureau of Labor Statistics, or USBLS, tallied only 4,800 working models in the country that same year. The field has shrunk since, with only 2,000 total models estimated to work in the US in 2021.)[10]

Then there are the long, irregular hours. Models report working fourteen- to twenty-hour days without advance notice, a practice so consistent it shows up in the USBLS job description: "Most models work part time and have unpredictable work schedules. Many also experience periods of unemployment."[11] The lack of scheduling predictability was also a complaint of warehouse workers I spoke to at a facility in Joliet, Illinois, who ship out clothing by the ton to Walmart and fast fashion chains. The practice is slightly more troubling in warehouse work, given managers' habits of locking employees into facilities during shifts, supposedly to minimize theft. Working long, irregular hours is of particular concern to parents, both in warehouses and in factories. In Cambodia, childcare options are few and expensive, so factory workers must delay having children, ship kids back home to grandparents, or invest in a good dead bolt and hope for the best during the workday.

For all fashion workers, the pressure to remain malnourished is high, although it is only one of many health and safety concerns in the industry. The 2013 Rana Plaza collapse in Bangladesh, in which more than 1,100 workers died, pointed to one common health crisis that plagues garment employees—dangerous working conditions. In Cambodia, mass faintings that started in 2011 and continue today point to another. Studies found that in the regular course of any given month, between tens and thousands of workers fall to the ground in a faint from a combination of undernourishment, long hours, heat, and bad air.[12] Workers in a Chicago H&M in summer of 2011 told me they left their jobs en masse when the AC conked out and they began to feel light-headed and faint in their store. Some H&M employees have access to company health insurance plans, although employees at other fast fashion outlets, like Mango, Zara, and Forever 21, do not. (In developing nations, health insurance does not often exist. Regulated garment factories are often required to maintain medical staff, but just as often will let that requirement, among many others, slide.)

Of course, the health concerns facing models are often less evident than indicated by mass fainting incidents: According to the Model Alliance survey, 68 percent of the workforce suffers from anxiety and/or depression. A quarter profess drug or alcohol dependency, and around a third lack health insurance. Undereating is pervasive: 31 percent of models admit to eating disorders, although the diagnosis as a mental-health affliction is called into question when undereating becomes a job requirement. Supermodel Amy Lemons was advised to eat only a rice cake a day.[13] Others are offered more subtle hints—often backed up by contract stipulations—to lose inches from hips, thighs, or rears.

Sky, former *Maxim* and *Sassy* cover model turned *Xena: Warrior Princess* regular, says the industry gave her PTSD. In an emotional YouTube video, she describes unsupervised foreign travel as a child and a lengthy shoot in a swimming pool, when her legs turned an unattractive shade of blue.[14] She was scolded for it, and years of such criticism began to wear on her, just as they did on Meier. Sky's emotional health tanked.

"The caste system on a set is specific and hard to navigate. And, while the model is the focal point, he/she is most often (unless she is a supermodel) at the bottom of the social caste," she elaborated via email. "The model must conform to what the makeup artist envisions for his makeup, even though he is placing his vision on her face. Same goes for the hairstylist and the clothing stylist. At each station, the model must fit into her role, even before she steps in front of a camera. No wonder most models I have ever met are so unsure of where they stand with anyone and always questioning, massively insecure. Because they are never offered any voice or source of security. Their body is a commodity for other people."

Emotional neglect, little sustenance, and unpredictable hours would create rough conditions for any worker under the age of eighteen, but the industry that sets the standards for beauty and desire in our culture is also a big-money honey trap for male predators. The poster boy for this ugly tradition is "Uncle" Terry Richardson, one of the highest-paid photographers in the world, who got his start at *Vice* before moving into couture and celebrities. He has been regularly named in sexual assault and harassment complaints since 2005, for on-shoot behavior including nonconsensual jizzing, offers to make tea from used tampons, and demands that models squeeze his balls. (It's hardly a surprise that Bill Cosby has evinced a strong preference for models in his long string of alleged sexual assaults, or that models' complaints were well represented amid the #MeToo onslaught of allegations.)

"This is an industry that obviously lends itself to sexual

harassment at the workplace," Sky tells me. But it's not just models and factory workers: big-box, name-brand retail and thrift-store employees as well as warehouse workers are also targets of verbal or physical aggression and unwanted sexual advances. One worker in the Joliet warehouse told me she was raped by her manager, fired when she filed a complaint, and reinstated only after several coworkers joined protests in solidarity. Other fast fashion warehouse workers say that sexual harassment at facilities is high because of the relatively few female employees and extensive surveillance equipment common in the foreign-trade zones where warehouses are situated.[15] (One might expect surveillance equipment to protect against worker abuse, until one realizes how easily the surveillants can find opportunities to commit such abuses themselves.) Even in supposedly sustainable secondhand fashion, the industry perpetuates the hypersexualization of female laborers: complaints have been filed against Apogee Retail LLC, owners of the for-profit Unique Thrift Store chain, for sexual harassment and abuse.

Model Alliance found that 30 percent of models experience inappropriate on-the-job touching, 28 percent feel pressured to have sex with someone at work, and 61 percent express concern over their lack of privacy while changing clothes. Only 29 percent feel they can report sexual harassment to their agencies, although two-thirds of those who have taken this step discovered that their agencies didn't bother to respond. 87 percent have been asked to pose nude without advance notification, which is a requirement for many agencies.

It's troubling enough to realize that models under the age of eighteen are routinely asked to strip for cameras without advance notice or supervision. But what makes the practice even more disturbing is that, in many cases, it's all perfectly legal. Agencies are able to recruit heavily from the preteen set thanks to a loophole carved out in the Fair Labor Standards Act of 1938, known as the Shirley Temple Act, which requires individual states to pass their own laws protecting child performers or farm workers. New York is one of many states that passed such protections—although eighteen others have not—and in late 2013, Model Alliance successfully petitioned New York to reclassify print and runway models under the age of eighteen as child performers. This category would assure that underage models can only work with state-approved permits and are entitled to limitations on the hours they work, while also guaranteeing them regular breaks, educational accommodations, and chaperones for those under sixteen. Compliance has been slow, but some in the industry say they've seen a slight upward trend in models' ages since.

There's a far more insidious ripple effect in play, however, when a culture sanctions very young girls as symbols of sexual availability. "Dressing little girls up to sell women's clothing affects the way women feel about themselves," Sky writes via email. "It affects the way men treat women. Why do we have such an out-of-control rape culture? Well if you look at the images of 'women' that advertisers are selling to us . . . [they] are of underage girls, cast as victims, their bodies taking on broken-doll positions, their eyes vacant, helpless, and submissive."

These images may demean individual models, but their cumulative effect also demeans the consumer, Sky charges. "How do you learn to memorize something? You repeat it over and over until it's in your subconscious," she explains. "It doesn't take advanced behavioral science to pick up the messages being sold to us."

Still, if you're the one selling the message, you might be able to make your individual peace with its pernicious content—provided the price is right. But here's another counterintuitive truth about the modeling profession: Models earn significantly less than you think. BLS suggests models in the US earned only around $19,300 in 2013, the year following the Model Alliance survey, which breaks down to a mean hourly wage of $9.28 per hour.[16] (This is about half the mean income in fashion photography that year, a male-dominated field where workers earn a mean of $37,190, and about one-fourth of the annual earnings for fashion designers, who also skew dude, and take home a comfortable yearly income of $78,410.) Retail-sales workers across all industries earned mean annual incomes that year of $21,890, with big clothing-retail chains claiming a workforce that's 85 to 95 percent women. Warehousing and storage workers, who tend to be male, earned an annual mean in 2013 of $29,630.

Look more closely at those earnings. The $9.28 per hour models earned in 2013 represented just 83 percent of the $11.50 per hour living wage in New York that year; while earnings tended to rise for models, the living wage did, too, and the gap between the two has widened significantly since then.[17] The most recent BLS tallies have models earning $31,910 per year, or 46 percent of a living wage, which is close to the same percentage of a living wage that factory workers take home in Mexico (48 percent) and in Bangladesh (41 percent).[18] It's true that part of a model's wages may be offset by the country-club lifestyle and, ahem, low food budget. Yet a percentage of a living wage is not a living wage: what stands out, across the spectrum of fashion-related labor, is that the pay for jobs dominated by women isn't intended to ensure survival.

Worse than low pay, however, is no pay. A 2013 report on Haitian garment factories found that every single one of the country's twenty-four garment exporters was failing to meet the national minimum wage, paying on average only two-thirds of what the law required.[19] Garment workers just outside of Delhi, India, who suffer gendered pay discrimination as a matter of course, have had unexplained deductions and delays in payment diminish their paychecks as well.[20] Indeed, workers at retail-outlet warehouses regularly face the range of practices known as wage theft. Laborers at a Walmart supplier in California, for example, won a lawsuit in 2014 for $21 million in back pay,[21] and workers at a Forever 21 warehouse filed a similar claim in 2013, stating that their bosses didn't compensate them for overtime, or provide them with meal or rest breaks on the job.[22] Garment workers in Cambodia, as we've already seen, fared no better during the pandemic. While brands like Adidas, Nike, Target, and Gap pulled in record profits, they failed to pass those profits along to workers—or in many cases, pay them back wages, overtime, or severance pay.[23]

Models have likewise reported that agencies dock pay over such offenses as having gained too much weight; it's also common, models claim, for agencies to delay paychecks for months on end.[24] Agencies charge for screen and other tests, visas, portfolios, delivery fees, etc.—all deducted from earnings before payout, and not always tallied for workers' financial records. Additionally, some designers pay in trade—apparel that is often too small to sell to anyone else and too flimsy to withstand the rigors of everyday wear.

"As we know, stuff does not put food on the table or a roof over one's head," Jennifer Sky elaborates. She's now left modeling for writing, but still sits on the Model Alliance advisory board and advocates for change in her childhood profession. "It is the extreme arrogance of the fashion industry that someone like Marc Jacobs, who runs a massive global corporation, would not pay twenty young women five hundred dollars each to walk in his show instead of 'gifting' them a garment or two."

But, as is the case with exploited warehouse workers, models face enormous structural barriers to getting their grievances heard, let alone resolved. Agencies guard against costly legal action by claiming that models are independent contractors, not employees. The temp agencies where warehouses contract for labor do the same. This designation leaves workers uncovered by many of the sexual harassment protections that apply to other classes of employees. It also just makes organizing difficult— and dovetails neatly with fashion's individuality-forward ethos.

"To offer no protections is absurd," Sky contends. That's why she wants to see her fellow models form a union. "We empower the worker who is selling us the goods; we too will become empowered. We make the fashion industry use adults to sell adult clothing; it will have a huge global impact."

♦ ♦ ♦

Modeling may rest on the shaky foundation we wave off as beauty standards, but its relentless reification of the self has far more distressing implications in a democracy than mere aesthetic preference would indicate. Models are not merely selected to reflect—read: entrench—cultural norms, but with every turn before the camera or on the catwalk, they're also empowered to invent them anew. The modeling industry strives to offer that unique combination of recognizably desirable and wholly inoffensive; models are charged to be serenely unattainable objects of beauty at the same time that they must remain studiously and generally unchallenging for the big spenders in white, mainstream, heteronormative America.

Racial discrimination is paramount. Meier, remember, initially excused the animosity she felt from other models because she wasn't competing with them for jobs. As a woman of color, she simply couldn't have put in for the same marquee gigs that her white counterparts would be offered; the industry is founded on the practice of physical discrimination. Meier's career path, she felt, was distinct from other (white) models'—even though the Supreme Court decreed in 1954 that separate but equal is not equal at all.

Designers seem never to have heard of *Brown v. Board of Education*—or if they have, it hasn't occurred to them that they, too, preside over an enormously influential institution devoted to educating American taste preferences. So it took more than fifty years before racial discrimination among models gained wider public attention. A 2008 *Vogue* article headlined "Is Fashion Racist?" prompted a burst of adverse publicity that had industry leaders swearing to beef up diversity practices in 2009, only to lose interest in the project again once the new spring colors hit the runway. Since the entire industry is virtually unregulated, no one seems to have proposed target numbers or quotas, and old patterns, in fashion, always reemerge. The number of Black models at New York's Spring Fashion Week hit a low in 2013, and the number of white models— 83 percent—a high, with some thirteen companies hiring no models of color at all.[25] By Fashion Week in fall 2016, the number of white models had dropped slightly to 75 percent—still not anything close to what a reasonable outside observer would call diverse.[26] When the *New York Times* tried to do a report on racial diversity in the fashion industry in 2021, only four of the top sixty-four fashion brands fully complied with reporters' requests for information. Sixteen more responded in part. Most of the rest declined. For its article on racial diversity in fashion, the paper of record was forced to rely on what the rest of us can see just as easily: that a majority of *Vogue* covers in the nine months before the article's publication date featured Black models. The single company in those top sixty-four brands the *Times* reached out to with a Black CEO was Off-White, whose founder/CEO Virgil Abloh died six months after publication.[27]

When I ask Meier, who is Asian European, about racism in modeling, her eyes widen. "It's part of the job," she says after a moment. "You develop a thick skin knowing you're going to be discriminated against because of your physical attributes and race or whatever anyway. You take it as part of the job."

Throughout our conversation, Meier had often paused to reconsider her experiences. Unlike Sky, she's not involved in the movement for models' rights, which helped to keep her replies from parroting any broader advocacy agenda. ("I come from the Philippines, where I don't think there are labor laws," she joked at one point.) She took a long pause here before continuing. "This conversation has opened me up to the idea that maybe some of these things aren't actually okay," she tells me. "But . . . they seemed completely okay. I accepted them. I didn't know that I couldn't."

Not knowing has consequences, of course, which is why the models' rights movement is important—although only as important as the movement for all fashion workers' rights. That, however, is substantial: by some estimates, between one-seventh and one-sixth of all working women in the world labor in some sector of the fashion industry, making it the field of commerce perhaps more responsible than any other for women's economic repression around the globe.

Organizing fashion workers has its challenges. We tend to see each workforce in this vast system as distinct to job description—models, retailers, warehouse workers, and factory employees each special little snowflakes, doing their part to keep consumers rebellious but stylish. However, each sector has more in common than it appears: the fashion industry submits its entire workforce to the same system of global Fordism that governs the race to the bottom in apparel manufacturing. The more the cutter and the packer are kept at separate ends of the line on a single factory floor, the less likely they are to communicate concerns about the factory they work in. Likewise, when factory workers are segregated from retailers, warehouse workers, and models, these related workforces are unlikely to collectively challenge the global garment industry's systematic disenfranchisement of women as workers and as consumers. For dressed in factory uniforms, sensible slacks, or glittery couture, women remain first-order targets of oppression as workers for the fashion industry—which targets them again as they line up to pay heavy markups in stores.

Still, organizing, even across Fordian divisions, within a single industry may not erase the core problems of fashion—or of modeling. "I don't know many models that have come out whole," Meier tells me honestly. "Not many come out of it feeling empowered, or confident, or having life skills to progress with anything other than their physical attributes. Models are some of the most insecure people I know. Period. And that's not healed by becoming a more successful model. That's healed by getting your ass out of it, completely."

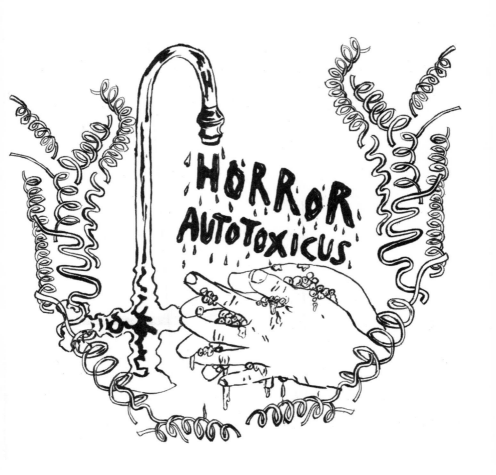

PAUL EHRLICH, B. 1854, D. 1915. The inventor of chemotherapy, helped create the first antiserum for diphtheria, cured syphilis. Developed methods for diagnosing diseases including typhus and tuberculosis. Foundational work in the fields of immunology, biochemistry, microbiology, neurology, and cancer research. Nobel Prize: 1908. Got a street named after himself in the Sachsenhausen district of Frankfurt in 1910. On a West German postage stamp in 1954. Commemorated with a crater of the moon in 1970. Several medical institutions, research laboratories, and even a human rights award are named in his honor. Odds are good that someone in your family history was snatched from the jaws of death by way of one or another of his accomplishments, which means that you might not be alive today without Paul Ehrlich.

Impressive CV, no? We call him a genius. (We call a lot of men geniuses.) What his many extraordinary accomplishments fail to point to, however, is his particular skill set, his unique and singular talent, the tic that allowed this solitary individual to develop so many medical advancements across so many seemingly diverse fields of science within one brief lifetime. The wellspring of his brilliance. What is it? For some it is math and for others an intimate knowledge of the heart or the mind. Not Paul Ehrlich. What he was good at was dyeing. Reduce his so-called genius down to one weird obsession and what you are left with is an indisputable gift for the application of color.

Imagine! It was dazzling. Otherwise Very Scientific Historical Accounts wax lyrical on the vials of powder stacked in his laboratories, hues left upon clothing, errant multicolored blotches on fingers awkwardly grasping the hands of more esteemed men in professional settings, men who did not begrime themselves in any direct way. Rich men. (Ehrlich's semi-embarrassed grin above that neatly trimmed beard.) We can look at it like this: he perceived the world in monochrome, the value of specific elements within it to be drawn out only by application of a compound of his choosing. A synesthete in reverse. Perhaps he will choose a methylene blue one day, a Bismarck brown the next, or an aniline red. Listen: *Iodine violet. Dahlia. Purpurin. Safranine. Fuchsin. Primula.* Words that describe hues so wondrous and variant that you have probably never seen them, too rare for even the rainbow.

He made color his thing. Took to carrying colored pencils around with him to elaborate upon his many genius ideas. On napkins at restaurants and on postcards in cafés and on tablecloths at home. (He married into the textile industry—of course he did!—and soiled table setting after table setting drawing depictions of side-chain theory or the impact of his antiserum on corynebacterium diphtheriae. Imagine the chortles of the houseguests as his wife cleared away yet another ruined linen; imagine their jokes! Lucky she had ample supply tucked away in her father's factories! Ha ha ha ha ha. Imagine her, laughing along. A doctor's wife. Polite, gracious. Raised by a man made wealthy by women's underpaid labor. Knowing that she had transcended that, at least that! But that her official contribution to history would still only ever be that she made the work of a genius possible. Imagine—remember—the smile of such a woman.) When Ehrlich ran out of linens, and postcards, and napkins, to what did he turn? The hems and shirt cuffs of audience members, his own clothing. Upon them all he developed his ideas about microbiology, biochemistry, infectious disease, human immunity—each wondrous, fantastic, and colorful in his depictions for guests.

But remember: it was only in the application of color to living matter that Paul Ehrlich was intellectually invested. The lightness or darkness of a color, the quantity of light reflected: we call it value. Value defines form and creates the illusion of space in the human eye. It is through a contrast of values that we define one object's separability from another's; by means of the gradation of value we perceive object mass or significance. What we credit as genius was Ehrlich's selection of the means by which to determine value. Don't ever forget that.

♦ ♦ ♦

Whether or not Paul Ehrlich himself matters and to whom has been a topic of no small amount of historical debate. Relevant to the dispute is the possibility that you may never have heard of the man until now, or have heard about him only as an associate of one of his better-remembered peers—Robert Koch, perhaps, or Sahachiro Hata or Emil von Behring—or have heard tell of only one of his many accomplishments. To you, perhaps, Paul Ehrlich does not matter so much. He may instead be your favorite-ever protomicrobiologist, and you wear T-shirts with his face on them every day. I don't know. To me he matters a great deal. Just not his accomplishments. It is his failures, vast and glorious, that I contend with daily.

There is no question that Ehrlich had fans—students, the public, other scientists—as well as grateful patients. When he first released his long-awaited syphilis medication Salvarsan 606 in December 1910 after extensive and careful testing, both the afflicted and the unafflicted (just to be "perfectly sure") wound 'round the block awaiting injection and, later, submitted appreciative correspondence until the end of Ehrlich's life.[1] Contemporary newspapers were less enthusiastic about his cure for the disease, then considered a plight suffered only by fallen women, so it rarely merited mention in print exactly what it was the new medicine treated. Salvarsan also brought out the scientist's first wave of dedicated detractors, who questioned the drug's safety and harbored misgivings about the cozy relationship between Ehrlich's lab and the pharmaceutical manufacturer that produced the substance.

Salvarsan was, yes, a new drug, and as such it was a vast improvement over the barbarity of the syphilis treatment in common usage at the time, liquid metal mercury, the injection of which directly into the bloodstream regularly caused organ damage and, slightly less frequently, death. But Salvarsan was also a new way of thinking about drugs. It combined two of Ehrlich's beloved catchphrases, *chemotherapy*—chemically derived treatments for eradicating disease—and *the magic bullet*, which referred to drugs that target disease-causing microbes without damaging host organisms. Salvarsan is a chemical compound that kills the spirochete *Treponema pallidum* or *T. pallidum*, the coiled microbe that causes syphilis, but at least in theory, nothing else. This made the drug innovative in function and in form, for Salvarsan also required a different way of creating drugs, and the 605 ineffective versions it took to create and release the successful 606th points to the intimate relationship between medicine and industry that Ehrlich spearheaded. The scientist retained a cut of the drug's profits, and a previous deal for diphtheria treatments that Ehrlich felt he'd been unfairly cut out of caused him to guard those profits carefully. (They would eventually be transferred to his widow.) It is also true, however, and remains so today, that when a medical doctor tells people that the only viable cure for a terrifying disease is extremely expensive, but is less open about his personal ownership stake in the sales of the drug, that people get skeptical.

One skeptic was named Dr. Richard Dreuw, a dermatologist by training who, by 1910, had taken a position as a doctor for the Morals Squad of the Berlin police. At a meeting of the Dermatology Society that year, Dreuw accused Ehrlich of releasing his dangerous drug after insufficient trials, despite that the five-month testing period was decried as needlessly overlong by physicians in the field of public health. Fellow dermatologists reportedly tried to quell Dreuw's outrage, and many of the more influential medical journals refused thereafter to publish his criticisms of Salvarsan and its inventor. For Dreuw, this was not a sign that his complaints were perhaps unfounded. Instead it signified that the whole of Germany was under the sway of a powerful Salvarsan Syndicate. When his assertions eventually cost him his post with the Morals Squad, Dreuw, it seems, knew whom to blame.

Dreuw was not the scientist's only adversary. He was joined in his outrage by one Karl Wassmann in

Frankfurt, publisher of a paper called *Der Freigeist* (The Freethinker), who also took issue with the financial machinations surrounding the drug. His more significant charge, however, was that the drug was being administered to sex workers without their consent and was killing them, which struck him as a basic humanitarian violation unbefitting a medical practitioner.

The gripes of the dermatologist and his publisher pal might have remained inconsequential asides were Ehrlich not Jewish and anti-Semitism not finding increasing foothold in Germany just then. But the detractors made friends in high places—like parliament, the Reichstag, and at the Basel newspaper *Der Samstag*, which would later inspire the National Socialist propaganda vehicle *Der Stürmer*. Fueled by hyperbolic praise in a Frankfurt publication comparing Ehrlich to Christ, *Der Samstag* took Ehrlich to task for the high fee for Salvarsan, claiming it was priced at an exorbitant seven to eight times the manufacturing costs of the drug.[2] Seven to eight times! Imagine finding a life-saving drug that cheap on the market today.

Four years into his campaign against the Salvarsan Syndicate, Dreuw—with support from the Reichstag—had built what we might now term a thriving platform. He used the momentum to request a national ban on Salvarsan from the Imperial Health Office, which he in turn used to demand a public debate on the drug. This debate was held March 10, 1914, and the offenses he charged Ehrlich with were many.[3] The most damaging was his assertion that 275 deaths over the previous four years were directly attributable to Salvarsan, as were, he suggested, numerous cases of blindness and neurological damage.

Ehrlich had ready answers for all charges, and more

than 130 different studies and papers on hand to bolster his defense. He described the precise charges and costs for manufacturing Salvarsan—statements he released in more detail later in print—and offered an explanation for those 275 fatalities, including those of sex workers. All of them, he suggested, alongside incidents of ocular and neural damage, were attributable to improper use. Salvarsan was a tricky substance, he explained, requiring cooled storage and freshly distilled water for dilution: some studies had revealed that physicians were skimping on both in the rush to administer a wonder cure for a painful disease that killed around three thousand untreated people in Paris that same year. Neosalvarsan, a less toxic version released in 1912, had already greatly reduced the possibility of physician error, and became the standard treatment for syphilis until penicillin appeared in the 1940s. But Dreuw was unconcerned with these more recent developments: Salvarsan had quickly become the most prescribed drug in the world, and did have its effects, both positive and negative, on the population at large.[4] More than a million people had been administered the substance in the four years since its public release. A mortality rate of .0275 percent—meaning one in approximately four thousand people at risk of death—is, still today, not unheard of for a prescribed medication. (Adalimumab, in comparison— sold today under the brand name Humira and prescribed for psoriatic arthritis, rheumatoid arthritis, colitis, and other autoimmune diseases—held a 1.165 percent mortality rate, or forty-four in four thousand, in clinical trials prior to release.[5] In 2016 Humira similarly racked up the most new prescriptions of any drug in the world, and it remained among the most popular medications prescribed globally until COVID-19 vaccines dramatically altered the stage of global drug prescriptions.)

The Salvarsan Wars, as the incident came to be known, were drawing to a close, and Ehrlich appeared the victor. Dermatologists the world over rushed to Ehrlich's defense to help secure the win. The Dermatology Section of the International Congress in London, for example, declared itself in favor of Salvarsan, and the Italian Dermatologist's Congress elected Ehrlich an honorary member that year when the group met in Rome.[6] Syphilis, a sexually transmitted disease then considered something of a public health threat, usually exhibits in its primary stage as a collection of sores around the mouth, penis, vagina, or anus. Perhaps its initial presentation as a dermatological blemish made the support seem necessary from the skin-doctor community, or maybe dermatology had at that point become so closely linked to the anti-Salvarsan brigade that various factions felt the need to clear the record. It's also possible that the specialists were responding to a subtext we can see clearly only in hindsight. Perhaps dermatologists did not want to be on the wrong side of the coming Holocaust?

However Dreuw's angry letters to various newspapers and journals seeking to defame Paul Ehrlich dog whistled the emerging anti-Semitic populace, marking the scientist with transgressions of blasphemy, blatant profit seeking, and public (read: Christian) endangerment. Banning the drug was one hoped-for outcome, therefore, but the failure of that project didn't change Dreuw's agenda: to eliminate Ehrlich himself.

The scientist died in August 1915. His dark, neat beard and full head of dark hair gone fully gray. The Salvarsan Wars had worn him out. Also there was his diet of mineral water and Cuban cigars. Can't have helped. Additionally there was that time he used himself as a test subject for a tuberculosis vaccine that appeared to have given him actual tuberculosis. At the age of sixty-one he had a stroke, and he died shortly thereafter. Topping his many accomplishments—the awards, the posts, the publications, the institutes, the esteem of colleagues—Ehrlich had cured syphilis. The scientist's legacy was most certainly assured.

♠ ♠ ♠

The fortunes of the widow Hedwig Pinkus Ehrlich seemed equally assured. She of the textile-industry Pinkuses. Born in 1864 to parents Josef and Auguste Pinkus. One of four children. She married Paul Ehrlich in the Neustadt synagogue in 1883 at the age of nineteen. The couple later had two daughters.

Josef's textile concern, damask-linen-weaving factory S. Fränkel Feinweberei in Neustadt, Upper Silesia, was at the time of the wedding one of the largest textile factories in the world. By the time Paul Ehrlich died, the First World War had stalled the booming table-linen business. Josef's son, Max, took over the concern after his father's death, but died himself in 1934. Max's son Hans then inherited the business and attempted to migrate it shortly thereafter, although this failed and the company was transferred to the heirs of Samuel Fränkel in 1938 under the Nuremberg Laws.[7] (Hans, Hedwig's nephew, emigrated to England the following year, where he died in 1977.)

The fortunes generated by the S. Fränkel Feinweberei, via the largesse of Josef Pinkus, provided consistent support to the Ehrlichs throughout their marriage, affording the scientist a private laboratory and giving him time for his early experimental research with von Behring. After the scientist came down with tuberculosis early in his career, he and Hedwig took two years to rest and recover in Egypt. The textile factory covered the family's expenses. Paul Ehrlich kept few autobiographical notes, and those he did keep rarely mention his wife (although the daughters make occasional appearances). None I have seen mention his father-in-law's economic support for his experiments, indeed his career in general.

Hedwig Pinkus Ehrlich would die in the US in 1948. A square-faced woman with wide, bright eyes and wavy hair tending to frizz. A photograph taken the year of her wedding shows a girl with an outsize head framed by a parasol, dressed in formal woolens at an outdoor tea party. Paul, seated to her left, is also young, dark haired still, and bearded, overly serious. But Hedwig seems amused by the photographer, by the meal, by the events, somehow satisfied. The damask table linen that cozies the outdoor scene is noteworthy. Remarkably little else about her is known. Even the online Pinkus-family-written geneal-ogy cites the glossy, fictionalized Warner Bros. version of her husband's career, *Dr. Ehrlich's Magic Bullet* (1940), as a primary source of information about her life.

How do women survive the deaths of their husbands? How do women live at all? What even are women? Histo-ries rarely offer insight, medical and scientific histories even less frequently. In textile factories today, it is nearly impossible to get by without a husband, a second income, a ride to and from work. Those who have not yet married cohabitate with other women to get by. Sometimes three, sometimes ten to a room. Spreading their mats along the floor in the crowded housing adjacent to the garment factories of, say, Southeast Asia. Waking before daylight to make a meager breakfast prior to the eight-hour workday, ten hours with overtime, more if the factory is illegal. Dinner differs from breakfast with the addition of a small amount of meat to the rice and vegetables, meat that has probably gone bad. Teeming with bacteria. Factory workers today regularly faint in mass numbers in the heat of the airless workroom as well as from malnutrition. Natural immunity to food poisoning is common, but not universal.

Presumably, Frau Ehrlich was above such concerns. She must have visited her father's factories, which would have looked much the same on the inside then as they do in Southeast Asia now: rows upon rows of machines invented to speed the labor of women, the women themselves barely able to keep up. The workers' anger at being partially replaced by unfriendly machines only increased as the age of industry advanced. The textile industry was the largest out-of-home employer of women in Germany before the First World War, as it is today throughout the developing world. From 1880 to 1890 the industry underwent rampant expansion. New inventions allowed for more small-handed employees, more workers crammed into small spaces trying to get more work done. What about toilets? Toilets were undergoing their own first surge of popularity in Europe at the time, but mostly in the homes of the rich. They would not come to Germany until the early 1900s. Why are we talking about toilets? You thought we were talking about sewing machines. Well, factory workers who are not given ample breaks in their workday to abandon their expensive machines must still relieve themselves. They went on the floor where they stood, long dresses allowing them at least the dignity of releasing water or waste in some privacy. Textile factories stank of human feces.

Certainly Frau Ehrlich did not shit where she stood, nor sleep eight to a room eating a small amount of rancid meat for dinner. But those are the material conditions of the industry her fortunes were first made from, the foundation on which Paul Ehrlich's career was built.

▲ ▲ ▲

In 1938 the National Socialists renamed Paul-Ehrlich-Straße, their first move toward expunging the Ehrlich name from the historical record. Hedwig Pinkus Ehrlich was forced to add a middle name—making her name Hedwig Sara Pinkus Ehrlich—to mark her as a Jew. It was this erasure of self-identity, a final cruel cherry on top of a sundae composed of rapidly diminishing wealth and an emaciated social circle, that precipitated her decision to leave Germany.

Formerly robust royalties for Salvarsan assured by her husband's shrewd negotiations had been cut off in 1921;[8] a legal battle reinstated a tiny annual payment in their place. The Nuremberg Laws, passed in 1935 but not enacted until after the 1936 Olympics, gradually stripped her and other Jews of an increasing volume of rights and freedoms, but for a while Frau Ehrlich had held firm in her belief that her husband's name and her familial wealth would protect her.

When both started to dissipate in 1938, Hedwig Pinkus Ehrlich emigrated to Switzerland, leaving behind most of her personal effects and all her valuables, commandeered by the Reich Chamber of Culture in Berlin. As was the law, she remitted nearly 90 percent of her remaining wealth to the state as a tax upon leaving the country. What she retained was later auctioned off, for which she received a small percentage of sales. She survived on the generosity of her husband's friends, although remember that these were friends her husband could not have made without the financial support of her father.

Frau Ehrlich stayed in Switzerland until late summer of 1941, when she moved to New York. The announcement of her stateside arrival on August 9 of that year was heralded by the *Chicago Tribune*, which devoted three paragraphs and a picture to the story, under the headline "Flees From Nazis." The item notes Ehrlich's invention of Salvarsan and quotes the widow decrying a "political situation which I could not tolerate." A colorful anecdote is supplied: As the Portuguese steamer *Nyassa* entered the harbor, the top mast of the ship hit the Brooklyn Bridge, cracking but not breaking. Frau Ehrlich and the other 689 European refugees—of whom we are to read her tale as metaphoric, if not emblematic—were visibly agitated. The story of these frightened immigrants was, more or less, this: foreigners in close proximity to brilliance barely escape Germany with their lives—finding respite in America!

Readers of the *Trib* would have been passingly familiar with Paul Ehrlich already, even if personally uncured of syphilis by his hand. *Dr. Ehrlich's Magic Bullet* had come out the year before, following on the heels of a popular movie about Louis Pasteur that had made the French biologist a household name. Starring Ruth Gordon as a beguiling Hedwig Pinkus Ehrlich, and Edward G. Robinson as the befuddled scientist, the film traded in drama and overlooked no small amount of factual detail. It got relationships wrong and simplified the science, and the item in the *Trib*, and others like it—for a few versions of the same story appeared in newspapers around the country, courtesy wire services—didn't do much to correct the film's errors. They did, however, fit neatly into a larger narrative, as did the film itself: that American entry into the horrible war was both justified and necessary.

From a certain perspective, it was neither. Roosevelt's December 7, 1941, decision was late coming, certainly, for humanitarian concerns about Germany's government had been publicly voiced since 1936. So on one hand, what was remarkable was that the US had been able to ignore what was going on under the Third Reich for five years. The American public had been staunchly against intervention when war officially broke out in 1939; public opinion gradually turned, a move in which media coverage played no small part.[9] When the Americans did enter the war, many argue the contribution was insufficient.

Regardless, most eventually agreed that something needed to be done, and the US needed to be a part of doing it. When the Nazis were finally ousted, no one complained that Paul Ehrlich's story had lost some nuance in all the hubbub.

Perhaps it would have concerned Hedwig Pinkus Ehrlich, had she not been scrambling for survival herself. It likely would have been easier for her to correct the record had her documents—her husband's notes, lectures, and papers—not been seized by the Reich. (Many remain unpublished still today.) Maybe she was just excited that her scientist husband was being revered in the US in a way he never had been in Germany, as a star, a celebrity.

Perhaps she was just aging, and tired, and no longer cared about nuance.

What happened, more or less, is that while the National Socialists in Germany were erasing Paul Ehrlich's legacy from the country, from history, and from medicine, the US propaganda machine was building it up stateside, cobbling rumors and stories together, many in translation, to create an image of a genius visionary scientist, unassailable, dedicated only to truth.

▲ ▲ ▲

About those failures mentioned earlier. Sometime during the early days of the twentieth century, Paul Ehrlich turned his attention to the body's natural defense mechanisms, devising a series of experiments that would eventually bring about Salvarsan 606 but which, in the meantime, established the framework for (mis)understanding the mysteries of the immune system.

On March 22, 1900, Ehrlich delivered a lecture at the Royal Society of London, a talk on recent findings titled "On Immunity with Special References to Cell Life." In it, he laid out his side-chain theory, a descriptive explanation for chemically specific receptor cells harbored to detect toxins and release antibodies. Although he'd been developing these ideas for nearly a decade, this lecture in English was the first time the theory received popular attention. Quite popular, in fact: this work led directly to his 1908 Nobel and the honorary title Father of Immunology.

To develop side-chain theory, Ehrlich conducted extensive animal testing. (He loved testing on animals.) Future generations would take him and the whole of science to task for that alone, and questions about how much empathy, and therefore emotional intelligence, can be employed during these tests do arise. Of course Ehrlich was injecting various animals with disease, and then various treatments for that disease that would fail on one or another front: either killing the animal with its own toxicity or failing to kill the disease with the lack of it. But that's just lab testing. Ehrlich was also injecting animals with blood and tissue from other, deader animals: the brain matter of a hog who had perished of one bacterial infection would go into a dog; the blood from a guinea pig who had successfully warded off another, shot into a cow. *Why not?* one can imagine Ehrlich thinking. *What's the worst that can happen?* Keep in mind that the scientist was not above testing drugs on himself. Whether he felt safe from harm or the practice simply gave him license to try out whatever occurred to him on others, we do not know. Anyway, experimentation is important to science and faulting him for making use of all that was available to him in the pursuit of scientific progress is not so much our concern. What remains important is how free he felt to do it.

Somewhere in these early days of the twentieth century, Ehrlich found cause to assign his assistant, Julius Morgenroth, the task of injecting animals with the blood of unrelated species in an attempt to foster the creation of hemolytic—red blood cell—antibodies. The two then attempted to immunize the animals with blood from others of their own species. Then with the animal's own blood. You see how this works? Why not. The animals are there for the taking, the lab equipment all paid for. (Staff photographs from the Charité, where the two first met, show Morgenroth, soon to become a bacteriologist in his own right, holding a rooster, standing next to a seated man holding a puppy. Interspersed among the white-lab-coated men are several other barnyard animals, some held too tightly to be captured by the camera. A guinea pig? Bird of some kind? All pulled from the lab to commemorate their roles in the advancement of science.) Over the course of these experiments, discoveries were made. While the animals tended to produce isoantibodies, or alloantibodies—antibodies produced by an individual that would protect against antigens, or toxins, coming from members of the same species, the mechanism that keeps some blood transfusions from being successful—the animals did not consistently produce autoantibodies, the mechanism in place in the autoimmune reaction that causes the body to attack its own cells.

The conclusions drawn from this observation are astounding. Instead of considering the possibility that the autoimmune reaction might be slightly more difficult to trigger than Morgenroth was at that point capable of, or acknowledging that what Ehrlich knew about the immune system did not yet extend to what might happen when that system turned on itself, the scientist decreed his observations to be universal, determined they would occur under all circumstances, held the force of a natural law. Autoimmunity simply didn't happen, Ehrlich declared—or more pointedly, that it might happen, but could not cause harm.

Something, he claimed, kept damage from occurring, some form of biological fail-safe like that employed by sippy cups and window guards. Ehrlich granted this mysterious mechanism the name horror autotoxicus because the man loved Latin. "Fear of self-harm" would be one translation, or "terror of self-poisoning." The general gist of Ehrlich's theory is that what keeps the body's immune system from attacking the cells of its own body is the innate corporeal awareness that an immune system turning on itself would be truly awful, a never-ending self-harm saga that might only cease with greater pain, disease, or death. Horror autotoxicus, Ehrlich explained, or the body's own fear of destroying itself, keeps the immune system from turning on its host.

What's most frustrating about this historic moment, besides its medical and scientific predominance, and the millions of other interpretations or considerations that could have entered into the picture then, is how clearly Ehrlich understood the basics of autoimmunity. He grasped how it functioned and what the damage might be. True enough, if the body's own immunodefense system were to attack the body's own organs, it would be awful even if endurable. Where Ehrlich was wrong, of course, was in the assertion that it did no damage. The most conservative of estimates places the current number of Americans with autoimmune diagnoses at twenty-four million. Others who closely track the diseases suggest that number should be doubled, that perhaps fifty million people in the US have figured out how to do on their own what Julius Morgenroth in the lab could not.[10]

Unfortunately, Paul Ehrlich's theory remained dominant for a hundred years, bestowed with the status of natural law. Horror autotoxicus was understood to be factual, and mounting evidence that autoimmune disease existed and did real damage to real humans was discounted until the end of the twentieth century. Even then doubts persisted.

Patients with rheumatoid arthritis through at least the 1970s often didn't bother seeking treatment; effective medications to manage the symptoms of multiple sclerosis weren't available until the 1990s. Individuals with Crohn's and celiac disease are still regularly told to ignore their symptoms for months or years in the hope that they will just go away.

For nearly a hundred years autoimmune disease wasn't thought possible. Of course, this caused delays in research and the development of effective treatments, and instilled the medical establishment with a basic distrust of patients complaining of symptoms. The fear that protected the body in Paul Ehrlich's imagination has instead inflicted greater damage upon it: what remains unknown about autoimmune disease today is so vast that we do not yet know what we do not yet know.

One thing that is known, however, is that women's systems go autoimmune approximately eight times more frequently than those of cis men worldwide. But we still don't understand why.

▲ ▲ ▲

We stand at a mind-bendingly fascinating moment in US history where we can begin to assess the full impact—positive, negative, and otherwise—of hundreds of years of the economic, political, scientific, and cultural dominance of cis men. Many of them—and forgive me if this is news to you—turn out to be horrible. Pedophiles, murderers, rapists, and psychopaths have driven some of the most compelling advancements of the modern era across all fields, and the narrow, bright light we have always cast them in is starting to fade. Figures no longer so harshly lit that only certain features can be discerned. We are all cast now in a hazier, more diffuse glow, past deeds as visible as current actions. If we can't oust a serial-rapist president, at least we know what he has done.

Is Paul Ehrlich as bad as all that? No. Come on. We can't place him among the Harvey Weinsteins of the world, the Charlie Roses, the Lorin Steins, the Roy Prices, the Louis C.K.s, the Matt Lauers. Those are just the names from media, the names of men we trusted to keep us informed of names in other sectors, but who didn't. Cancer researcher Inder Verma, geneticist Francisco Ayala, neuroscientist David Sweatt. Everywhere are men with outsize power who wielded it primarily for personal gain and only secondarily subjugated mass numbers of women. Wait— if that is the measure, then maybe. Maybe Paul Ehrlich is as bad as all that.

He was certainly a little odd. I mean, besides the cell-dyeing thing. He subsisted, we know, largely on mineral water and thick Cuban cigars, often tearing through more than a box of the latter per day. Admittedly that is no crime. These boxes he carried about with him, grasping them in his hands more tightly than even his various records, documents, and papers, which he often lost in cabs or in his office, under other pieces of paper, never to be seen again in the onslaught of information balanced precariously on every surface in sight. His cigars were precious, and he would not let anyone else touch them, not even people who are paid to carry things to and fro, people like porters and manservants and delivery boys. He is said to have interrupted his extremely important work on more than one occasion when there was concern that the lab assistant he sent to pick up more cigars might not be up to the task. According to his biographer Martha Marquardt, who was also his housekeeper, Ehrlich received deliveries of at least twenty-five Havana cigars per day, at strengths so delirious that visitors to his home couldn't stand smoking them and passed when offered. Ehrlich smoked continuously throughout the day, and wouldn't loose his grip on the box of them he carried when he traveled.

Ehrlich was obsessive, perhaps monomaniacal. At one point he asked a younger colleague out for a celebratory drink, which the colleague had taken to mean wine. Ehrlich ordered a mineral water for himself, then talked so obsessively about his own ideas that he never once ordered anything for his guest or, for that matter, offered him any of his mineral water.

Maybe it's a small offense, in keeping with his befuddled-genius-scientist reputation. But one gets the sense from reading Marquardt that Ehrlich was something of a self-absorbed, spiteful beast with little impulse control. She tells a tale, transcribed from one participant in a letter to her, of a trip Ehrlich undertook with two companions on a train. Having denounced a detractor at a conference—Dr. Ludwig Pfeiffer, and not Dr. Richard Dreuw, for even a shallow dig into Ehrlich's career will unearth more than a few disputants—quite publicly, and theoretically already having proven both the merit of his own work and the lack of merit of his opponent's, Ehrlich became incensed on the train, remembering Pfeiffer's arguments and yelling about them at the top of his lungs. Although the porter returned three times to ask him to remain quiet so the other passengers could sleep, and finally threatened to kick them all off the train, Ehrlich couldn't stop shouting about the man, who, presumably, had already been thoroughly denounced.[11]

Marquardt writes of it all as if in the thrall of a petty necromancer. She is going for an aura of Stendhal syndrome, but her prose instead carries a whiff of Stockholm. She describes scenarios in which Ehrlich walks into a room and barks a new order at her, which she dutifully complies with, and records faithfully out of glowing esteem. These descriptions include situations such as Ehrlich leaving off dictation and wandering around the room for fifteen minutes to conduct various experiments that just occurred to him, without bothering to explain what he was doing or why, or failing to locate her a chair when he wanted to work in a room that didn't have one free. (He would never clear papers away for her, nor for any other reason, and would not allow her to touch his papers either.) He often interrupted the dictation of one letter with dictation for several other letters but, as Marquardt says, would not take clarifying questions. She was left to her own devices in figuring out whom Ehrlich wished to say what to, exactly.

Maybe that was okay with her. I don't know. I'd find it annoying. But what shines through her description is the degree to which the man consistently failed to register or respond to the discomfort of others. Certainly this can be conveyed with a wink and some charm in the biography of a renowned scientist. But it becomes less acceptable in, say, the examination room of your general practitioner.

Indeed it is when Ehrlich was practicing medicine that his befuddled tendencies seem most immediately destructive. In 1878, the twenty-four-year-old Paul Ehrlich was granted an assistantship at Berlin's famous Charité hospital. Just a pup! An inveterate dyer. The man who understood that chemical compositions could be seen in vivid color. He'd barely graduated, skipped most classes, and skated by on the strength of his pursuit of knowledge about dyeing things, and somehow landed this job. He was, let's be honest, kind of a fuckup. And here he was, at the famous German research hospital, one of the only healthcare options for folks of no means. Folks who would accept more experimental treatment because it was the only treatment they were likely to get.

German physician Friedrich von Müller started there, eventually becoming something of a protégé of Ehrlich's. He's commemorated by Müller's sign, the official name for a throbbing of the uvula at the back of the mouth that heart-damaged patients exhibit during systole, when the heart refills with blood in the course of its normal pumping efforts. In his memoirs, Müller gives an account of the obstetric wing at the Charité, and Ehrlich's mentorship. "What we most dreaded," he writes, "were obstetric duties, for only a few of us doctors at the Charité had acquired sufficient practice in midwifery."[12]

Müller goes on to describe the late-night rousting from bed by the night nurse, urging him to the obstetrics ward with some birthing-related emergency. And the medical advice he'd received from his mentor Paul Ehrlich: "If you are called to this ward," Müller writes that the great man had told him one day, "carry on washing and disinfecting your hands until the department medical officer returns."[13] Müller's sad recollection is that occasionally the medical officer failed to return, and he was forced to help a patient in great distress himself.

It's unclear what sits most uneasily about this description: Müller's clear discomfort with female patients (whom he also fails to credit for, you know, helping in the project of childbirth) or Ehrlich's handy suggestion for skimping on medical duty, a practice we can assume was tested by Ehrlich himself. Women giving birth in lying-in hospitals in Europe died in childbirth before the 1880 advent of antisepsis measures at rates of about eighty-five in a thousand,[14] meaning that eight or nine of every hundred patients Ehrlich avoided tending with a feigned, sudden interest in hygiene would perish.

Did any die while Ehrlich stood washing his hands, hoping someone else would take on the unpleasant task? What was he thinking while he stood there, scrubbing out his multicolored hands? Was it, *Entire bodies bore me, I sure wish I had a microscope right now*? Or, *Please don't let them notice me, I am going to be famous someday but feel no obligation to ensure that actual human lives in front of me are saved*? Or, *Women? I have more important things to do with my time*?

Or was Paul Ehrlich only ever thinking, *I am the important one here, the one who matters. I am the one who determines value.*

CONSUMPCYON

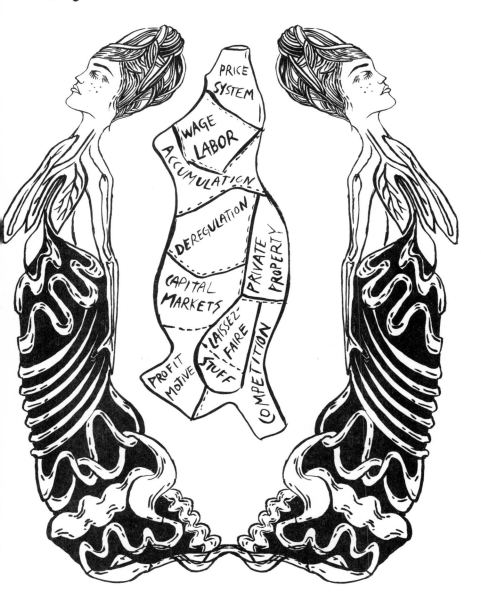

MARIAN IS A BRIGHT young woman living in Toronto in the mid- to late twentieth century, an employee at a small market research firm who spends her off hours juggling an attractive but hard-to-please boyfriend, an irresponsible roommate, a tittering gaggle of officemates, and unenvied friends stuck in the baby-making grind. She is well educated and able-bodied, and filled with all the hopes and dreams a woman could imagine for herself before the second wave of feminism took hold: marriage, she supposes, to a man, and kids, maybe, eventually? Friends to entertain, certainly, in a nice home, although come to think of it, Marian isn't entirely sure what she wants. In fact, Margaret Atwood's 1969 novel *The Edible Woman* (Atwood herself called it "protofeminist") is primarily concerned with what Marian *doesn't* want, and how her disinterest is culminating in physical symptoms. Marian, a product of—and an important cog in—consumer society, eventually finds herself unable to consume. "This is ridiculous," she says to herself when she first encounters problems with food.[1] What, our protagonist wonders frequently, could possibly be wrong with her?

Atwood is short on details of Marian's life before her digestive issues arise, toppling with them the character's status as able-bodied: the book opens with the entirely forgettable sentence, "I know I was all right Friday when I got up," the kind of banal, normative statement the able-bodied wish to be able to make once sick. The author is stingy, too, with elements of Marian's person, as well as with precise descriptions of her emerging ailments. Still, there are plenty of words between the opening sentence and the appearance of Marian's consumptive failures some 170 pages later, and many of them, upon close inspection, reveal themselves to be cleverly feminized alarm bells. As Marian grows increasingly concerned about her inability to eat, she becomes alienated from her own body—reflected in a shift from first to third person narration between the two halves of the book—and increasingly unable to articulate her concerns: she stops being "all right" sometime after Friday, but because Marian never verbalizes her concerns, the reader doesn't have any clues as to when she gets sick or what form her illness really takes.

What we gather about Marian in the first half of *The Edible Woman* is that she is white, Canadian, upper-middle class, and professional—"normal," we're given to believe, if a bit reticent to contradict the insufferables that surround her. Her character is filled out in the negative: she is "not a blonde," she disapproves of her roommate's drinking habits, she backs away from conversations about child-rearing. Marian desires not to bring offense, clearly, but Atwood designs her inoffensively: she is Everywoman, that literary device into which Atwood's largely white feminine readership might slot themselves. In the common parlance, Marian is "relatable."

Yet Marian's apparent normality is a large part of the trouble, for there is no visible manifestation of her problem with food. She does not develop a tumor, for example, or appear alarmingly frail to any of the other characters in the book, nor does she gain weight. As the adage goes, seeing is believing; not being seen, therefore, leaves one at risk of not being believed, although Marian offers no explanation whatsoever for why she can't eat, so is in no danger of being discredited. The reader only ever knows that, to Marian, the problem is quite real. Yet without any detailed symptoms, the reader has no idea if the problem is biological or psychological.

A "refusal of her mouth to eat," the ailment is named at one point, the blame for her disability placed on "whatever it was that had been making these decisions, not her mind certainly." Her jaw fails to open, she cannot lift her fork, she is hungry but finds she cannot take a bite: Marian has been diagnosed by successive decades of readers as vegan, anorexic, nervous, allergic, hysterical, and a victim of our hyperconsumerist environment.

It might be more to the point to diagnose her, simply, as a proto-Everywoman—and although Atwood's visionary status most popularly refers to her later works, ailments remarkably similar to Marian's have become quite common in recent years among relatively young North American women. The American College of Gastroenterology estimates that 10 to 15 percent of adults in the US have irritable bowel syndrome (IBS), for example, although only 5 to 7 percent have received a diagnosis. The symptoms and concerns of this disease are as vague as Marian's, and therefore it is just as difficult to diagnose. Alongside dozens of autoimmune diseases—many with food aversions of little understood biological or psychological provenance—IBS has, in the more than fifty years since Atwood first envisioned something like it, become a modern epidemic.

▲ ▲ ▲

ANNE ELIZABETH MOORE

Marian's troubles arise one night at dinner with her fiancé, Peter, when she can't finish a steak. Her standard diet of TV dinners, packaged puddings, and boil-in-the-bag entrees often leaves her craving something freshly made, so she rarely leaves leftovers when she goes out. Yet she can neither clean her plate, nor offer any reasonable explanation to Peter for her sudden lack of interest in the meal. Although she keeps up appearances in the coming days, her difficulties only worsen.

"The day after the filet, she had been unable to eat a pork chop," Atwood writes. All meat is out. Soon Marian finds she can no longer stomach a growing list of foods: next is dairy, and shortly after that, vegetables. Her primary concerns are social, for she continues attending parties and dinners, but resorts to hiding food whenever she cannot finish it. The third person narrative voice further confounds readers seeking details of the protagonist's digestive troubles, and it becomes difficult to trust Marian's description of events as accurate.

The novel ends tidily, in a too-neat domestic scene in which Marian symbolically offers herself up for consumption but, rejected, ends up symbolically consuming herself. Deeply rooted social norms—like that convenience food is harmless, for example, or that single women crave marriage to eligible bachelors—are overcome *like that*; Marian is cured. She can eat again and, newly single, can offer her symbolic self up for other men to eat too. Marian is back on the market, as it were: Atwood's joke about Marian's reentry into consumer society.

It reads false, and as we will soon see, it is false, at least for the millions of women in North America who suffer ailments resembling Marian's. Yet on all other fronts, the book is unusually prescient, even for an Atwood novel. For *The Edible Woman* is not merely a story about consumerism, about the body's need to eat as biological phenomenon and as cultural metaphor. It is a story about broken political economies and their impact on the physical self.

Take the difficulty in diagnosing Marian, for example, which comes from her seemingly normal existence. She works in advertising ("market research") and intends to marry a good-looking young lawyer. Obviously she is surrounded by brands and thinks about how they might fit into her life for a good part of every day. She considers ads, and whether she likes them, even outside of the office: she has internalized her role as a consumer so thoroughly that she is apt to have a product for dinner that she worked on during the week. Her friends are bearing children—both in and outside of wedlock (although those who start outside of it quickly want in). Her future, in other words, seems clearly planned.

Unfortunately, Peter, her good-looking-young-lawyer fiancé, has no positive interpersonal attributes. He is dismissive of Marian, and the sex they have is perfunctory and passionless. He enjoys hunting and then describing the animals he has killed over dinner. He is a bore and a letch, but it is unclear how much of this Marian can perceive because her behavior is either predictable for a character written before the 1970s—she defers to him more and more over the course of the book—or inconsistently written, which is unlikely, since Atwood tends to create characters with rich interior selves. The reader experiences the friction between the two potential explanations for Marian's submissiveness through a simmering rage, an experience common to gender-aware readers of works written before the second wave of feminism. At the time, of course, marriage represented one of the only paths to financial security for women, aside from being born rich. (Women in the US couldn't have credit cards in their own names until 1974.) So readers won't be surprised that Marian pursues marriage, even with a partner she occasionally acknowledges is imperfect. Financial security is necessary to lead the well-branded life she clearly desires. Marriage is not something Marian finds negotiable.

Yet something is wrong. That Marian's entire life trajectory is thrown into question when her consumptive issues arise is one clue that the book is about far more than mere consumption, but the *New York Times* missed it in its 1970 review:

> As her wedding day approaches, Marian quite literally begins to lose her ability to consume things. First she rejects steak, finally she cannot even stomach salad. A case of bridal jitters, says a married friend. Or, as I think the author means us to half-seriously see it, a piece of truth-telling dementia that is a symbolic answer to lying sanity. Not to eat or be eaten up like a confection of calculated flavors might be her heroine's unconscious aim and Miss Atwood's symbolic sense.[2]

The thesis that consumerism is the entirety of the problem that Atwood means to point out likely held a certain logic—maybe even an unwashed allure—when the review was published. (A tried-and-true revolutionary of the 1960s once told me that, by the 1970s, he had believed capitalism was over. It seemed clear to him and his colleagues, he said, that culture had reached peak consumerism. Then he laughed.) The onset of Marian's ailment, however, isn't a reaction to food itself, nor the infiltration of ads, brands, sales pitches, and jingles into her world. Her revulsion is triggered instead by an awareness of how it all works together, a glimpse at the man behind the curtain and what he's preparing for her back there.

Marian is not, in other words, symbolically oversatiated by the array of products on offer. As her body prepares to reject beef for the first time, she is watching her fiancé carve his steak at dinner. It reminds her of an image in a cookbook, a butcher's diagram of where the various cuts of beef come from on a cow. "She could see rows of butchers somewhere in a large room, a butcher school, sitting at tables," Atwood writes, "clothed in spotless white, each with a pair of kindergarten scissors, cutting out steaks and ribs and roasts from the stacks of brown-paper cow-shapes before them."

The image keeps her from finishing that particular cut of cow, but she soon stops eating pork and sheep too. What rankles her is not solely that meat is flesh: it is that an entire system is devoted to keeping her from realizing that meat is flesh, a well-regimented design incorporating safety scissors, clean uniforms, and dotted lines, all in place to ease and conceal the elaborate machinery that turns living bodies into food. Consumption is not distressing her, nor the culture that facilitates it. Instead, she is repulsed by the economic and political systems that create them—marked more by the factory, the uniforms, and the workers than the presentation of cows as meals.

Nonfiction food writer Michael Pollan describes a similar scene in *The Omnivore's Dilemma*. At the meat counter in your local supermarket, he suggests, "you encounter a set of species only slightly harder to identify" than in the produce aisle, where foods tend to retain something of their original form. "The creaturely character of the species on display does seem to be fading," he notes, as more and more the animals on offer for consumption "come subdivided into boneless and bloodless geometrical cuts."[3]

But who is doing the subdividing? What Marian's body begins to reject is the contraption that offers up these geometrical portions. The friendly face of industrialism hides the assembly line not only from the consumer (Marian), but also from the consumed (the cow, whose drawn-in facial expressions on the butcher's diagrams make it seem perfectly content with its role in the proceedings). Of course, these two roles are fungible: "Every time she walked into the supermarket and heard the lilting sounds coming from the concealed loudspeakers she remembered an article she had read about cows who gave more milk when sweet music was played to them," Atwood writes. "But just because [Marian] knew what they were up to didn't mean she was immune."

Therefore it's not totally wrong when Marian's married friend attributes her stomach troubles to wedding jitters— the "piece of truth-telling dementia" noted in the *Times*. For marriage is simply another stage of the assembly line's conveyor belt to which Marian feels strapped. *The Edible Woman* also predicted correctly that feminist sci-fi of the era to come would liken hell to a reasonably happy marriage to a businessman or tenured professor, replete with kids and a dog. Joanna Russ's *The Female Man* (1975) draws such a comparison; *I, Vampire* by Jody Scott (1984) contains a harrowing nightmare sequence in which a morally ambiguous character's death results in an imagined, horrific afterlife of baking, child-rearing, and hubby coddling. As Marian plans her wedded life, she may well be stepping onto the pathway toward a dystopic Stepford-wife future. (Ira Levin's *The Stepford Wives* was published only three years after *The Edible Woman*.)

Yet Marian isn't balking exclusively at marriage itself, or even just marriage to charmless Peter. At one point following their engagement, she finds him acting inscrutably, and she imagines he must have purchased a marriage guidebook, to match the camera and legal manuals on his coffee table. "It would be according to his brand of logic to go out and buy a book on marriage, now that he was going to get married; one with easy-to-follow diagrams," she thinks. She uses loving words, but soon her body is rejecting her placement on this assembly line too.

What triggers Marian's illness is her glimpse of the elaborate system she feeds into and from, a multiuse machine with a myriad of moving parts, all of which push different aspects of her life toward a single end goal. Her every move, consumption inclusive, has been predetermined, and her clothing, relationships, and even reproductive goals (she is annoyed to discover) selected for her in advance. It makes Marian sick. Atwood doesn't name the system her protagonist glimpses, but we now know it's called capitalism.

♦ ♦ ♦

In the early part of the new millennium, Rachel was a midtwenties pharmaceutical graduate student in Kansas with three dogs, three cats, and a fantastically attractive boyfriend named Alexey. Rachel is quite pretty herself, with long, dark hair; clear skin; deep, dark eyes; and a strong, sincere smile. Like Marian, Rachel's planning to marry soon, but she's been having some digestive issues, and managing them is taking up a lot of her time.

Luckily her boyfriend is patient and supportive, even when their dinners together make her outrageously ill. She and Alexey are particularly fond of a certain frozen pizza, as Rachel writes in a 2009 post on her blog. "In the past, I have gotten some heartburn from it and definitely a ton of gas build up, but it's never made me sick. Last night was the first time it did."[4]

Her story, instructive in its detail, continues. After she finishes eating, Rachel writes, "My stomach felt extremely bloated." She shifts position, then stands, but nothing will relieve the pressure in her gut. "Then out of nowhere came the urgency," she writes. "The feeling of needing to get to a restroom with no time to spare is horrible, and experiencing it out of nowhere in a crowded place or somewhere you can't leave quickly is terrifying."

Rachel goes into some detail regarding diarrhea and nausea—she's got a fear of vomiting that makes the latter particularly unpleasant—and expresses gratitude that she was not only able to get through that pizza night without throwing up, "but also that I only had to take GasX." Other brands whose products she cites would be immediately recognizable to her readers, many of whom suffer similar symptoms (Pepto and Imodium are her go-tos), as would the cycle of illness she describes:

> I hate it so much when foods I've eaten for months with no problems suddenly cause me to have an episode. I had just said to my mom earlier that day that I thought I was finally regaining control of my life and not living it in fear

of what food was going to hurt me and make me sick again. All I ate today was cereal because I didn't want to get sick again. I am so sick of cereal. Just when I think I'm in the control, my body steps in to remind me how much of a joke that really is.

Rachel's tale of pizza-related torment was published four decades after *The Edible Woman* was released. Although her story has much in common with Marian's, she doesn't mention the book. The only thing she mentions reading on her blog is her own blog, which she uses to catalog her IBS. It isn't a platform for self-pity, however; her blog offers the public service of community building. Commenters regularly leave notes on this post, about pizza and IBS, as well as on her other posts, which may be about diet, drug regimen, the social anxiety of living with this particular disease, planning a wedding with a chronic illness, or plain old poop. Rachel blogged approximately once a month for seven years, and her readers often leave notes to thank her for writing, or briefly describe their own similar stories. ("Reading your blog post, it honestly sounded as if I was reading one of my own journal entries," one writes.) Commenters frequently note how desperately they have been searching for stories that reflect their own experiences. (One example: "My sister has been dealing with this for the past 2 years and people really have no idea just how much of an issue it really is. It totally changes your life!")

Irritable bowel syndrome is hardly rare. A relatively common diagnosis given to folks that experience discomfort in the large intestine, including cramping, abdominal pain, bloating, gas, diarrhea, and constipation, it's something of a catch-all diagnosis, bestowed upon sufferers with symptoms but no recognizable disease (although IBS does often evolve into something more clearly defined, like ulcerative colitis). You may not even know if your friends have it: as may be surmised, propriety keeps the diagnosis from coming up in most polite conversations. Internet discussions, therefore, which offer both a degree of anonymity to sufferers and, presumably, the comfort of writing from a controlled environment, frequently result from Rachel's posts, although her blog is not the only one to tackle IBS, nor the only one to do so from a personal-narrative standpoint. Others offer insight into recipes, drug regimens, new treatment options, fitness routines, legal advice, or other aspects of living with IBS. (There is, for example, a now-defunct YouTube channel devoted to toilet jokes from someone going by Positive vIBS Tribe.) There were, in the early two decades of the new millennium, countless blogs by people who suffered a range of gastrointestinal disorders and autoimmune diseases— *Ali on the Run* looks at marathon training with Crohn's, for example, while *ChronicBabe* covers a wide range of chronic illnesses.

Reading such blogs offers a glimpse into the suffering of what the National Institutes of Health (NIH) estimate to be almost twenty-four million Americans afflicted with auto-immune conditions.[5] (Another eight million, the National Institute for Environmental Health acknowledges, have autoantibodies that indicate a potential for autoimmune disease, while the Autoimmune Association, formerly the Autoimmune Related Diseases Association, used to perhaps more correctly point out that these numbers may underestimate the preponderance of autoimmune disease by about half.[6]) The primary struggle of the afflicted (like

CONSUMPCYON

Marian's) is to understand why their bodies have betrayed them, and to do so, input from other sufferers is required. Even the least talented writers have dedicated readers and commenters, so community seems to be forged not around talent, but out of sheer desperation. Most blogs are kept by women, who make up approximately 80 percent of the diagnoses of autoimmune disease worldwide. From a labor perspective, we should note that the keepers of such sites probably aren't getting paid for blogging, or are at best offsetting site update fees (in the tens to low hundreds of dollars per year) with ads, so most of the work of blogging could be described as the unpaid emotional labor of creating resources for a community that cannot find sufficient help anywhere else. Whether or not bloggers have day jobs may also be relevant: it is notoriously difficult to have the most common autoimmune diseases officially recognized as disabilities and receive social-service benefits, despite the inability of sufferers to consistently meet the demands of day jobs. Let's situate this, too, in the context of a capitalist—as opposed to consumerist—society. The work that Rachel and other first person chronic health-ailment bloggers do fills a medical need for patient-focused conversations currently untended to by privately funded, profit-driven healthcare systems, which consistently defund support groups, online chat spaces, and counseling services that could provide similar. Nor is the need addressed by the rising tide of wellness centers, leaders, or products, all of which tend to prize notions of purity and health that the chronically ill by dint of diagnosis cannot achieve (not to mention their exorbitant costs!).

That symptoms just as mysterious as Marian's would

become common in the decades that followed *The Edible Woman*'s publication was certainly unforeseen. But because mysterious feminine digestive troubles and invisible ailments have started to gain medical recognition in recent years, they have lost some of their comedic bite. In fact, "half-serious," "dementia," and "lying" are only a few of the pejorative descriptors the *Times* lends a scenario in which a woman can't simply eat whatever is put in front of her. It is only through the steadfastness of Atwood's pen, it seems, that we refrain from considering Marian a wholly unreliable narrator. "People suck, in general, when it comes to accepting and respecting IBS as a real issue," Rachel writes in one blog post.[7] I'm apt to let her speak for the millions of other sufferers of understudied diseases: Today, people with similar symptoms are often passed from doctor to doctor for several years—the most-cited average is seven—before receiving a diagnosis. Many have watched as their symptoms are written off as psychological—the medical-industrial complex version of the *Times*' "lying."

The problem, however, might not lie in millions of women's heads. A 2001 study at the University of Maryland found that although women in general have lower thresholds for pain than men, and tend to experience it for longer, their symptoms are often treated less aggressively.[8] More recent studies have suggested that greater nerve density or variances in hormone levels in the female body deepen the intensity of negative physical sensation; some studies have shown that folks who transition experience less pain as they begin taking testosterone. In emergency rooms, women wait for pain medication an average of sixteen minutes longer than men and are 13 to

25 percent less likely to receive an opioid medication. A separate study in the *New England Journal of Medicine* showed that, among cancer patients, women were significantly less likely than men to receive adequate treatment for their pain.

Researchers remain baffled by these findings, although Diane E. Hoffman and Anita J. Tarzian told lifestyle news outlet *Mother Nature Network* in 2015 that they'd come across a handful of recurrent explanations in interviews with medical staff. These include presumptions about men being able to manage pain better and not complaining about it until it is "real"; some women's ability to birth children, which is thought to imply an ability to manage any amount of pain; and women's presumptive tendency to exaggerate and complain instead of describe sensation accurately.[9]

The world of medicine, in other words, tends not to believe women when they say they are in pain, which in the realm of invisible illnesses like Marian's is often the only symptom on offer. Fold in a host of known food-related disorders—anorexia, bulimia, etc.—and we can detect a general cultural tendency to label women's problems with food as little more than psychosomatic, mere psychological issues undeserving of deeper study, never thought to be exacerbated by external or environmental forces, or indeed to be provable in any way.

Marian never describes the full range of her bodily failures, either to another character or via interior monologue. It's a trick of Atwood's, to force the reader to believe a female character's version of events in order to follow a story line. It also saves the character from the embarrassment that millions of other women have experienced, of

being told—by acquaintances, loved ones, and doctors—
that their illnesses are all in their heads.

▲ ▲ ▲

You've heard of celiac disease, a diagnosis given to two to
two and a half times as many women as men, in which the
body's immune system attacks itself when triggered by
the ingestion of gluten. Perhaps you've even reposted one
of many articles claiming to debunk the wheat protein's
link to physical discomfort on social media—a sharable,
friendly way to discredit women's pain.

However much the precise mechanics of the relationship between certain foods and autoimmune disease may
not be understood, foodstuffs beyond gluten have been
linked to certain autoimmune responses. Usually, autoimmunity is considered a medical mystery: for unknown
reasons, doctors say, the body's immune system turns on
itself in the same way it would attack a parasite, virus, or
other foreign invader. The resulting inflammation causes
pain as well as physical impairment. Yet some health practitioners—naturopaths, in particular—root autoimmune
disease in food sensitivities.

Several food-elimination protocols are therefore
suggested for the autoimmune: some name-brand, like
the Paleo diet, and others more tailored to individual
responses, like the low-FODMAP diet (to cut down on
short-chain carbohydrates), elimination programs (to identify problem foods), low-histamine diets (to quell allergic
responses), and rotation diets (for those who can't identify any specific food relationship to symptoms beyond
ingestion). Such diets, however unreasonable they may

sound to those who have not tried them, do tend to work for a large number of people.

Yet despite extensive anecdotal evidence, scientists have been slow to look into a relationship between consumption and autoimmunity. The reasons for this are likely myriad. While many might tend to blame Big Pharma's exclusive focus on profits for the holdup, it may equally be due to the gender of the majority of sufferers. Although medicating illness is profitable, there are surely enormous profits to be made in staving off illness, if the price point for continued health is set high enough. It seems more likely that the tendency of the sciences to overlook autoimmunity is rooted in the low numbers of women in STEM. Women chemists, for example, make up only 40.4 percent of the field, and women chemical engineers only 25.9 percent, according to career demographics tracker Zippia. Nor are there enough women funders to ensure such studies take place: Less than 15 percent of the 2022 Fortune 500 CEOs are women. (None as of publication are openly trans or nonbinary.) The persistence of the gender wage gap means that women do not currently have the economic clout as a class to fund or demand such studies. Anyway, those who perceive a clear need may be too ill to mount a campaign, or already wrapped up in the sustaining care work of blogging.[10]

Only recently, therefore, has a connection been proven between food and these poorly studied ailments. A June 2015 report in the peer-reviewed journal *Autoimmunity Reviews* found that common food additives contribute to intestinal leakage, which creates the conditions for autoimmunity.[11] The specific trouble-causing additives named in the report—all used under the claim that they improve taste, appearance, or the shelf life of food—include emulsifiers, glucose, gluten, organic solvents, microbial transglutaminase, nanoparticles, and salt.

Authors Aaron Lerner, a professor at Technion – Israel Institute of Technology, and Torsten Matthias, of the Aesku.Kipp Institute in Germany, suggest that these additives contribute to the breakdown of intestinal walls—a condition commonly called leaky gut syndrome—from which the autoimmune response can follow.

The report cites the rise in autoimmune disorders—many diseases have three times the number of diagnoses that they did four decades ago—that are primarily occurring in nations with high rates of processed-food consumption. Also noted are the specific disease categories with rapidly rising numbers of diagnoses (neurological, gastrointestinal, endocrine, and rheumatic), as well as the geolocations of the diagnosed, which seem to indicate that environmental, and not genetic, factors are the primary reason for the uptick in these ailments. The report describes a corollary rise in the use of food additives, intended to increase "the world's capacity to provide food through increased productivity and diversity, decreased seasonal dependency and seasonal prices." (In Brazil, for example, the years 1987 to 2003 saw a 46 percent increase in the intake of processed food in the average household. Virtually unheard of three decades prior, within a decade of the introduction of processed food to Brazil, rates of rheumatoid arthritis stood at around 1 percent of the population and incidents of psoriasis at 2.5 percent.)

To recap, the seven additives listed above are now being found in more foods. Those foods are eaten in more households around the world. And bodies in those households

CONSUMPCYON

with previously healthy immune systems are becoming dysfunctional. Causality, Lerner and Matthias warn, has yet to be proven—the report only indicates that these particular food additives contribute to leaky gut syndrome, from which the autoimmune response follows. "Precise mechanisms responsible for the development of nutrient-induced autoimmune disorders are unknown," the authors contend.

Still, recommendations based on these findings are in order, they say. Patients with family histories of autoimmune disease are recommended to limit exposure to these additives. Additionally, strengthening FDA nutritional labeling standards—policies that have been designated barriers to trade by lobbyists and are being modified or dropped entirely[12]—and further studying the impact of food additives on immune systems are equally strongly recommended.

What this means is that individuals may be going autoimmune due to personal consumption habits. Yet autoimmune diseases in general—their worldwide spread, their increasing diagnoses, and their worsening symptoms—are likely triggered, at least in part, by the far-reaching machinery of globalized food production.

▲ ▲ ▲

A food industry reliant on additives to ease its own spread throughout the globe has become central to a socioeconomic system based on private ownership of the means of production. McDonald's stands as a shining example. In the decades since *The Edible Woman* first appeared, the chain has been documented using food-preparation techniques from farm to table that are questionable at best and extremely dangerous at worst, exists now in outposts formerly hostile to Western presence, and—Marx would be impressed by the company's allegiance to his definition of capitalism—exploits the workforce to such a degree that fights to raise the minimum wage to fifteen dollars per hour have been commonly sighted at the burger chain. (The company had just opened its 1,000th restaurant and was about to expand into all 50 states when *The Edible Woman* came out; today the company's own website claims over 38,000 restaurants in more than 100 countries in the world.)

Pollan describes a visit to McDonald's in *The Omnivore's Dilemma*, where he muses on the poultry-like meal his son orders. "The most alarming ingredient in a Chicken McNugget," he explains, "is tertiary butylhydroquinone, or TBHQ, an antioxidant derived from petroleum that is either sprayed directly on the nugget or the inside of the box it comes in." A form of butane, Pollan notes, that causes vomiting, collapse, or worse, TBHQ is lethal in very small doses.[13]

The mainstream food movement in which Pollan plays a significant role has given us a contemporary understanding that the standard consumption habits of the Western world can be quite damaging to consumer health. Of course, there is also a disease *called* consumption that in the nineteenth century killed as many as one in four Brits. Susan Sontag traced its earliest usage to 1398 in *Illness as Metaphor*. "Whan the bode is made thynne," writes John of Trevisa, "soo folowyth consumpcyon and wasting."[14] Consumpcyon was the common name given to tuberculosis, a disease that at one point was as mysterious and misunderstood as autoimmune diseases are today. Mysterious, but ever present: the ill were described as languorous, hollow chested, romantic, and pale. They appeared to be in the process of being consumed.

It's a markedly different metaphor than can be applied to the autoimmune, who have less a disease in the traditional sense than a consistent internal dysfunction. However much autoimmunity may be triggered by food consumption—and despite the fact that many patients can control the negative effects of these disorders to at least some degree by restrictive diets—the autoimmune are not being devoured by any malevolent outside force. The bodies of the autoimmune attack *themselves*. In some cases, yes, eating away at them over time, but the immediate symptoms of inflammation occur at the site of self-generated attack. In fact, what is markedly different about autoimmune disorders as opposed to any other public health crisis in history is that the whole language of fighting disease does not apply. The body must instead be soothed into remission, must learn to lay down its weapons entirely.

This is the logic behind restrictive diets, that certain foods—and food additives—trigger attack more than others. This isn't an explanation that makes much sense to medical professionals, however. Doctors who don't outright laugh when asked about connections between autoimmunity and food are few; others are more tolerant, although one often gets the sense that one is being humored. ("There are people who feel better when they don't eat certain things" is a common medical response, if an unhelpful one.) There are only a handful of doctors in the US, however, who believe food to be a primary trigger of autoimmune disorders that aren't situated in the intestines, like rheumatoid arthritis, lupus, and psoriasis. Even Lerner and Matthias's groundbreaking studies on leaky gut syndrome have been slow to filter through to the medical world.

In some ways, the reluctance of the medical profession to acknowledge that disorders suffered by one-fifth of the US population are partially triggered by modern food production is understandable. Recent changes to the global supply and processing chains were made, as Lerner and Matthias acknowledge, to increase nutritional access and limit hunger. Admirable goals, to be sure, and certainly one could argue that slight suffering among the few is a reasonable price to pay in pursuit of increased health for the many. Yet such a justification can only hold for so long before changes become necessary to restore public health. Incidence of type 1 diabetes rose 64 percent between 2001 and 2017, according to the *Journal of the American Medical Association*,[15] and to significant effect: autoimmune diseases as a class are said to shorten a patient's life span by around eight years.

Some have also found symptoms worsening and triggers increasing in number. Celiacs who have trouble managing their symptoms, for example, have begun in recent years to avoid dairy as well as gluten, which some suggest is an indication that dairy proteins have begun to mimic the wheat protein. Others, already diagnosed, are simply accruing more diseases at a seemingly unstoppable clip, regardless of how well their original symptoms have been controlled through standard food-restriction protocols, a possible indication that more foods predict or trigger the autoimmune response than is currently suspected. On several concurrent fronts, the negative effects of globalized food production seem to be quickening at an alarming rate.

Marian solves her problem with a symbolic gesture: a small cake replica of herself that is offered for Peter's consumption. He doesn't want it, so she eats some—a miracle!—then offers the rest to another man. It's a joke about consumption. Who has the right, and obligation, to consume? The joke is on Marian, for she must be consumed, however symbolically. The unremitting inevitability of consumption is, of course, capitalism. Yet the joke is also on women like her, on real-life women like Rachel. For Marian's symptoms went away following no medical intervention. Perhaps it was all in her head after all? The reader is left to wonder.

Not all readers, of course: millions of women around the world know that their bodies are failing not through any mental or emotional flaw, but because the system under which they live is causing damage. They feel it as clearly as Marian did. Today, bodies regularly grow intolerant of production lines, global distribution, and decisions made with only profits in mind. Like Marian, women throughout the industrialized world are no longer capable of consuming what is on offer. Their bodies, too, are rejecting capitalism.

A FEW THINGS I HAVE LEARNED ABOUT ILLNESS IN AMERICA

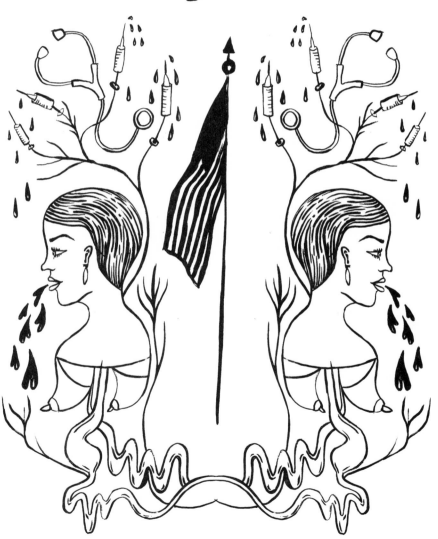

1. Sit with a friend through cancer treatments because you love them, not because you believe they would do the same for you. They won't. Cancer changes people, and it makes people vulnerable. If your friend survives, they will want to reinvent themself. They will *need* to reinvent themself. What I mean is: your friendship is probably over, once your friend beats cancer. You will help them do that—survive—but your only reward is likely to be that knowledge. You may, later, go through cancer treatments yourself. It is possible that you will do this alone. Even if you sit with three different friends through cancer treatments. What is important to realize is that you helped them survive because you are good at survival.

2. Your best doctor is your body. My hope is that you will find other doctors who have more training in and experience with illness than your body does, but I would not count on it. Weigh professional opinions and theories against how a medication feels in your palm, or what comes to mind as it digests in your stomach. Avoid processes that allow the administration of treatment to get too far away from your own hand. Not because you should not trust other people—you should—but because it matters if you shake before you give yourself an injection, or if your heart aches every time you go in for new lab tests.

Another way to say what I mean: notice what makes you feel bad, and avoid doing it. I have found that most people do not know when they feel bad. I personally did not learn how to tell when I feel bad until I turned forty-four.

3. Many people will offer advice. No—everyone, in some way or another, will offer advice. Some will tell you to change the way you eat, or how to feel. They may suggest you find a better doctor, as if you do not live daily with the failures of modern medicine or the limitations of your own practitioner. Others will tell you how you can make it easier for them to understand what you are going through, or demand that you be patient with them. You must try not to laugh. If people grow upset at your behavior, they may repeatedly ask what is wrong with you, even after you have told them one million times that you are sick. Still others will believe resolutely that you have done something wrong. They will say, "Aha," at the wrong moment as you relay an anecdote, or forward articles to you about smoking, yoga, or drinking tap water. They believe they do this out of kindness, but what is being said is: You are failing to live up to my expectations. I am being let down.

If you bother to listen to other people at all—although I can understand why you would not—you may wish to translate everything anyone tells you into the phrase "I care about you more than I myself realize, more than I am currently capable of expressing." Do this without speaking, inside your own head. It is only for you.

4. This is important: do not hate your disease. If you can, try not to hate anything at all, but that may prove too difficult. You have a right to be angry. Still, hate is for people who feel they have nothing to lose, for people who are comfortable sitting in judgment of others. Also, hate takes time and energy. Time you could be devoting to far more important pursuits, like laughing at jokes, or research. Hate only inspires more hate; what you need right now is love.

5. Mass disabling events, unfortunately, do not concern the US government, nor do they represent anything more than annoyances to the major corporate forces that seem to guide federal policy. Acting as if a public health crisis does concern our government, presenting information as if it could be convinced to, or otherwise behaving in a manner that presumes you may be cared for by people whose salaries you pay, and in many cases whom you have elected to public office, is futile.

6. Protect yourself emotionally, perhaps more ardently than you are now forced to protect yourself physically. Try not to engage in situations in which your health can be pitted against someone else's interests, as in asking someone to refrain from smoking in your presence, or working at a job during a surge in an ongoing pandemic. You will be forced to remove yourself from the situation to protect yourself, of course you will, even if this propels you into other dangers. Even the smoker or your boss will understand this, in theory. Perhaps you have briefed them on your needs on a previous occasion, and they have claimed to understand them, your

needs. You cannot expose yourself to the potential of smoke inhalation or to the coronavirus. You have stated this clearly, and it is true, and now you must maintain your boundaries. Even if it leaves you without a ride home, or unable to afford groceries.

Yet the smoker or your boss will argue with you, in a friendly or a not-so-friendly way. They will say, "Oh, I will just blow the smoke over here," or, "Wear a mask." They might say, "What is your problem, we are outside!" or, "The inconvenience that accommodating you would cause to me is too great."

This, be aware, also causes damage. It is toxic when someone expresses to you that their convenience is more important than your health. It stays in you forever. From that moment on, you understand that every single person you meet may—probably does— secretly believe that your life matters less than their agenda, less than their habits, less than their comfort. This is why it is important to do everything in your power to avoid having to tell someone, "What you are asking me to do could make me sick, or kill me." Refrain as best you can from raising your death as a point of negotiation.

7. When someone discovers you are sick, do not be surprised by their antipathy. For example, someone may say, "Oh, my grandmother committed suicide when she was diagnosed with that!" Or an acquaintance might give you false information about your disease. This will happen, surprisingly frequently, with doctors. Friends in media and entertainment will write you into stories as a character, taking your hard-won

experience of survival from you without permission and using it to advance their careers. You may see yourself become a morality tale for hard living, dangerous choices, sexual promiscuity, eating meat, lack of religion. You may find your high school best friend does this, or your auntie. It is what people do: use what they come across for their own purposes. You cannot blame them, but you do not have to be around them.

Alternatively, you may meet someone who claims similar ailments. They may express sympathy for you, or seek to discuss the peculiarities of their diagnoses over intimate dinner parties. You may bond. Yet do not be shocked the day they excitedly explain that their doctor has pronounced them cured of an incurable disease, or fully recovered of something from which one simply does not recover. Possibly, they will excitedly relay the means of their recovery to you and claim that positive thinking, or prayer, or a diet of red meat cured their ailment, but they will be wrong, and this will depress you. It may have been an enormous relief to you, to have made a friend who understands what you are going through, to have met someone that you thought you might be able to call in a real emergency. The loss, to you, may be real, even if the illness was fabricated. These were efforts expended to be in your company, yes: manipulation, misrepresentation, opportunism, all employed because someone desired your attention. Perhaps this is flattering. But these efforts represent something more troubling too. A lack of comprehension of a disease that may be quite damaging to you. A very basic ableism that allows some to claim and then to dismiss diagnoses at will. The idea that sickness is a choice, and the implication that you have chosen wrong.

Another acquaintance, after a frank conversation about your illness, may comment, "Wow. It's terrifying that such a thing could so easily happen to me!" Laugh at that person. Laugh at their narcissism, at a worldview that holds that illness picks and chooses victims for a moral or ethical reason, or any reason at all. Laugh at the fact that they feel safe when you know that they are not. Hope that they remain safe because an unjust comeuppance for narcissism is illness. But do not trust that person. Do not trust anyone who takes from you in your moment of greatest need.

8. Others will avoid you. *Most* will avoid you. They do not want to deal with mortality, yours or their own, or what strikes them as worse than death: frailty, weakness, disability. This will make you deeply sad for the world, and for yourself, that you may never speak to your best friend again, to any of your best friends again. If you ran a company or organized events in your neighborhood, people whose lives you worked hard to support may not gather around you.

Let me tell you this because no one else will: people are awful. I am sorry that you will feel alone much of the time. I am sorry for every doctor's appointment and bad-news phone call that you will endure by yourself. I am sorry about the time that pharmacist was flirting with you until he looked at the drug you came in to pick up and paled. I am sorry that an insurance agent once called you to demand $986 to pay for the test result that indicated a $1,200-per-injection drug prescribed by your doctor had given you a new disease. I am sorry that you will regularly show up at gatherings of your closest friends, of people who claim to love you, and be the only one in a mask. I am sorry for the bitch on the bus who couldn't see you were in pain so she complained loudly for three miles that you wouldn't give up your handicap seat for her shopping bag. I am sorry that the energy you once spent making others laugh or dressing up for parties or planning elaborate adventures is now used to fill weekly pill containers, do tai chi, visit specialists, and try to stay awake.

I am sorry it seems so easy for others to forget that you are important.

9. You may live long enough to watch those who treated you poorly when you first became ill become ill themselves. Perhaps they suggested your illness was not real, or undermined your attempts at improving your environment to better respond to your needs, or devalued you on the basis of diminished physical function or limited emotional availability. It does not take long for others to grow sick. Only a few years, tops. Sometimes months. A person who abandoned you upon diagnosis reveals that they must start cancer treatments; another who criticized you for the manner in which you performed illness is hospitalized with mysterious symptoms. The most self-aware of these individuals will contact you and apologize for their previous behavior. They will ask for your support, now that they understand. You may consider giving it to them. Remember that you needed their support several years ago, but you managed alone; at the very least, you

needed them to refrain from maliciousness, although they could not stop themselves. Now they are asking for your good wishes, your love, your hard-earned wisdom, but what they want even more than that is for the slate to be wiped clean, to never have harmed another person simply because that person was unwell. It is what they think about while they sit for endless hours with chemicals pumping through their veins, what keeps them awake at night in the ward when all the other patients are resting. But guess what? People hurt one another.

Will you forgive them, allow them back into your life knowing that their request for forgiveness is pure egocentrism, that they have learned nothing from their initial mockery and later accrual of illness, that they are just scared of dying? Or will you be the one to remind them how deeply abandonment can hurt, how it can change you, and how you can survive it? I have no idea. Your call.

10. Very rarely, certain people might react to your illness by saying effortlessly: "What can we do, your community?" It may take a year to hear this question, or longer. You may think you will never hear it. In truth, you might never hear it. You will expect to hear it when you post on Facebook about a negative test result or mention to a small group of friends over coffee that your doctor is concerned. The crucial question will not come then. It may not come when you fail to show up for birthday parties, although it is clear that your absence has been noted. It may not even come after a week when you cannot answer the phone, or when you do not have

the energy to respond to emails. When you effectively disappear from the face of the Earth.

You will be made aware then that people are gossiping, but you will also be aware how few of those asking others about you have ever asked you how you are. Everyone will feel that they have expressed concern and wished you well, but the actual number of people who will do so is quite low. You may see, in other words, evidence of community forming, but it will still take time for its benefits to be offered to you.

Try not to sob when this happens. The friend who finally mouths these words will believe they are the hundredth person to say, "What can we do? How can the people who care about you show it?" Do not mention that you don't know if you believe in community anymore, or tell them the names of community members who have hurt you beyond repair. Do not test their faith in the power of people to gather in support as yours has been tested. Just answer their question.

11. Your European friends will make what seem to them to be very logical suggestions: Request a paid leave from work, go to a health spa for a month, begin receiving disability compensation. Supplement your Western medical treatments with high-quality and easily accessible Chinese medicine. These treatments may not be affordable or in some cases available to you in any way. Your European friends will be baffled by the barbarism of the State. It will not make sense to them how a rich nation can so severely take advantage of its population. This is important: do not attempt to answer their follow-up questions because a whole lifetime can be

wasted describing the injustice you are currently experiencing. It does not need to be yours.

12. If you happen to be chronically or terminally ill when a pandemic strikes, consider throwing your television, computer, and telephone out the window. Do not go to the library to check Twitter. Do not ask friends who come over for coffee what's happening on Instagram. You should probably cancel subscriptions to all newspapers and magazines. If you are in the unfortunate position to share social circles with public health experts or politicians or op-ed columnists, refuse all dinner invitations, even if everyone promises to mask, vaxx, test, and triple booster. I can tell you now what you will miss out on: hours upon hours upon hours of people who claim to care about you agreeing as a matter of public policy that your life is expendable.

13. Even if you have been assured the most basic of care by federal law—however minimal indeed for those whose diseases are little understood in the first place, and for whom there are therefore no effective treatments—you may suddenly find yourself in your doctor's exam room crying over the threat of its repeal, sobbing at changes in your eligibility for treatment, wailing about the lack of affordability of care. You doctor may face personal threats from the same administration: perhaps she was born in a country from which others have been denied entry to the US by surprise executive order, or fears annulment of the law that allowed him to enter a same-sex marriage with his partner of several decades. Certainly your doctor faces a potential job loss if you

and others are suddenly ineligible for their services. Your doctor may also cry. However, it is possible that your doctor could say, "I have a plan." Then your doctor may detail the black-market prescription dispensaries, back-alley lab testing facilities, medication alternatives to in-person procedures, and unsanctioned exam rooms nearby that will allow you to survive. You may wonder if this is a movie, or a trap. The sliver of hope, however, will buoy you. Let it.

14. You will learn to get by on very small kindnesses. These are often gifts so tiny they mean nothing to those who dole them out. A fruit basket sent by the secretary of a man you worked with once, whom you have never met in person. He is an acquaintance of a good friend who never contacted you after you received your diagnosis. A heartfelt but single-line email from a colleague on the other side of the country; an extra-warm hug from someone you respect but do not know very well; an angry email from someone in your same line of work, someone who rightly tells you to buck the fuck up when you have professed a desire to give up, someone who does not mind that you are sick but cares enough to see past that and spots that you are about to make an irreversible mistake. Over the course of a month, you may experience only one such event, or you may not experience any at all after several years. But if you are granted such a kindness, and you thank the person who administered it later, they will not remember what they did. They will have no idea that they saved your sanity or your life, that collectively and without even trying, the people who have thoughtlessly supported

you have created a world that you are desperate to stay in for just a little while longer, no matter how difficult.

15. I'm going to be honest with you. I have no reason not to be. I do not know you, and we may never meet, but I can say without a doubt that your doctors may not be telling you the truth, and your friends certainly aren't. Drugstore clerks honestly do only want your money. RNs have plenty of other patients set to take your place. Your company can do without you just fine. Your pets will even move on. (I am not saying that people do not love you. They do.) Yet a moment of horrible honesty is required, so here it is: there is a chance that you will not make it through this, whatever "this" is for you. You may die soon; you will certainly die eventually.

Peer at that statement. Ignore that it is sorrowful and unkind, even as you admit that it is true. Take it as a reminder to care for what you love, and a plea to be courageous in defiance of unspeakable cruelty: of the State, of the system, of disease, of community, of individuals. If you do not make it through this—whether it is this virus or this economy or this political regime or this side effect or this policy change or this diagnosis or these very, very difficult days—let us remember you as someone who loved very deeply.

Do not let us forget how much you cared.

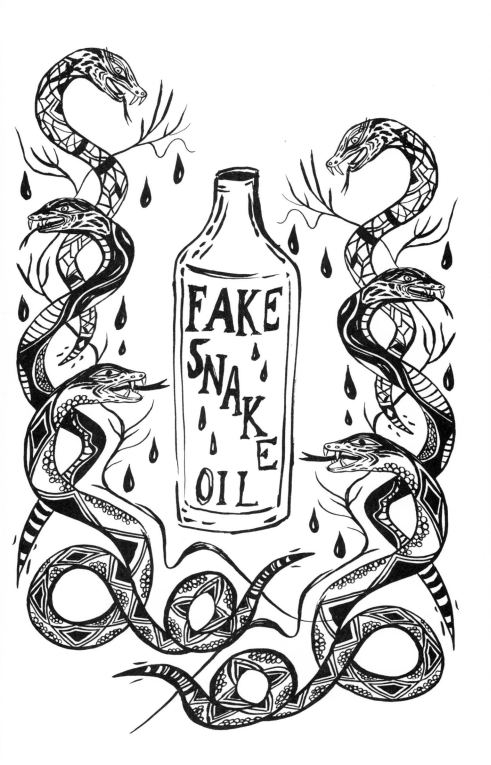

THERE'S A CITYWIDE yard sale going on in Marfa, Texas, about seventy-five miles north of the US-Mexico border, and what's for sale, mostly, is baby clothes. The teen-pregnancy rate here is rumored to astound. A backlash, one imagines, against the cold inhumanity of the Minimalist occupation that moved into town after artist Donald Judd first did in 1971. Also for sale: interestingly rusted tools that won't fit in my backpack, books of the how-to, cooking, and joke varieties, and wholly inappropriate items for June in west Texas: wreaths, fake snow, holiday lawn ornaments. Inside someone's home behind the row of tabled goods, someone boils a pot of beans. It smells like warm protein and onion.

I am drawn to a table displaying a collection of bottles enigmatically labeled "1.50 ALL." They are confusing for reasons beyond whether the price is per piece or by collection: the containers are new, and each bears a dot-matrix-printed label falsely touting a folksy curative. One, for example, is a rejiggered Newman's Own salad dressing bottle, still bearing the signature plastic screw cap, while two others contain liquids that had resolved genuine medical ailments before their recasting, now, as fake medicines. The various back-bedroom quacks conjured to respond to imagined concerns, and the potions not, in fact, created by them in the long-ago prospectin' days include: Abel's Dysentery Powder, Mrs. Smith's Finest Headache Drop's [sic], Clark Stanley's Snake Oil Liniment, and Gus's Pure Liver Tonic. Nearly all of them also bear an image that seems to have been scanned in at a breathtakingly low number of dots per inch: the caduceus, or the staff of Asclepius—commonly recognized as the "medicine symbol," a snake or two entwined around a rod—but we'll come back to that.

Under this serpentine mark—of authenticity, natch—are listed each potion's "ingredients." The label for McQuirre's Joint & Leg Cramp Formula with Quinine, for example, states, "Ingredients: Salt Water," and indeed, a ring of salt deposits crowd the cap, and the air wafting from it tastes mildly tinny. The liver tonic is made with a stale-smelling "Grape Juice," while the rheumatism-and-body-ache rub claims "Mineral Oil." Abel's Dysentery Powder, should you find yourself with a make-believe case of that bloody diarrhea symptomatic of a potentially deadly parasitic or bacterial infection, is said to contain "Flour." The bottle labeled "Pure Smelling Salts" is in fact filled with a floral-scented "Bath Powder"—an interesting substitution, given recent findings that bath salts contain a chemical linked closely to MDMA or ecstasy, and men who've confessed to snorting it have reportedly chewed off major portions of other men's faces. Even more interestingly, the pungent bottle labeled "Marshal's Skin Easement Soak" is said to contain "Smelling Salt."

♦ ♦ ♦

Borders are ever present in Marfa. Between the Latino and white sides of the segregated cemetery; between art-tourist destinations and the feed stores and refrigerator repair shops that are so clearly indicative of daily banal needs for two separate economic and social classes. There is also, of course, the local border patrol.

Borders within Marfa are patrolled by language— not just the Spanish-English divide, but by the varying connotations of vocabularies specific to differing social, professional, age, and gender groups. Local teens, when they're not out impregnating one another with abandon, derogatorily call the recent wave of artist whites "Chinatis" after one of two foundations established to uphold and expand the legacy of the minimalist Donald Judd. (When they *are* out impregnating one another, they sometimes do so at the Chinati Foundation, where a vast field is filled with Judd's concrete boxes, one of the few public spaces in town to offer any privacy.)

The older Latinos in town display ambivalence toward "outsiders," another local name for the recent cultural immigrants who are primarily white. For their part, the "outsiders" behave as occupiers: they form community among themselves, pitching in and working on behalf of "the locals" when a governing body calls upon them to do so, but remaining largely, perhaps deliberately, unaware of the predominant culture of the region. Wikipedia, a site frequented by regular internet users who have graduated from college and, according to a Pew Charitable Trusts report from 2011,[1] tend to earn greater than $50,000 per year, lists the racial makeup of the city as over 90 percent white and less than 7 percent Latino. A local business site, however, perhaps more accurately suggests that Latinos make up almost 70 percent of the town and white non-Hispanics less than 30 percent.

In other words, what you believe to be true about Marfa entirely depends on where you stand in relation to what border. Still, the town smells the same no matter where you find yourself: like hot dust and a bit of hay, tones of wet concrete, maybe, after a rain, and a constant base note of flat, stale beer.

▲ ▲ ▲

The enigmatic price quoted turns out to refer to all as a *group*, and not all as in, *all of them are the same price*, so I happily hand over a dollar fifty to the yard sale proprietess without further consideration, explaining to the brown-skinned woman at the card table that my mother kept snake oil bottles over our kitchen sink.

She cheerfully pulls two more glass containers out from under the table and asks if I want them too. They're leaking, and she says, "The labels are getting all messed up." I don't catch her gist, considering that she has clearly typed them up on the computer herself, made superfluous use of the modern fonts Old-Timey and Cowboy Narrow Condensed, and slapped them on whatever just-used glass bottles she could find lying around. Most are topped with a plastic not even available until the mid-1980s. The illusion of authentic snake oil isn't maintaining itself in the first place, so there's not really a lot here to "mess up."

But she shows me: stuff has escaped the bottles, and the labels are becoming difficult to read. "They're broken," she says in a moment of laughing honesty. In a decision I now view as wholly arbitrary, I decide that the purchase of broken glass bottles filled with fake cures for real ailments goes an unreasonable step beyond the purchase of glass bottles that will still cure nothing but have remained, so far, intact.

"Better not try to cart them onto the plane back to Chicago," I tell her.

"Oh, you're from the Midwest?" she asks, my personal snake oil salesperson. I catch a whiff of her perfume; it is cheap and sharp, which I like. High-end perfumes tend to seduce, aiming to blend in as if a situation could exist in which a person's neck might naturally have rubbed against a rare out-of-season flower. "Be sure and tell all your friends back home that they really take these down in west Texas," she tells me. "That they really work."

She guffaws, but she's not exactly joking. I suppose that going in on a laugh together at her region's expense is preferable to what she may see as the alternative: that I will laugh at her expense later without her permission. In fact, I don't think the collection of cures I've amassed is funny at all. They're far more authentic than their creator seems even to realize, and I thank her for them profusely. This only seems to confuse her.

♦ ♦ ♦

The master narrative about unlicensed medical practitioners is that they are fakers, liars, true capitalists. That they take nothing and spin it to their advantage, sucking in the trust and faith of the unwitting masses for personal, extravagant gain. That they do not discriminate, and are therefore not swindlers or standard con men, who will work a target over a stretch of time, twisting your personality quirks into their profit. They create instead a basic view of the world and its ills and your role therein. And they sell, simply, a tincture necessary to your survival within it, provided you are able to follow—or, less strenuously sometimes, simply trust in—the worldview they describe. There is nothing personal about what they do: their audience self-selects. They're called charlatans or mountebanks, or sometimes chiropractors, witches, medicine men, doulas, yoga practitioners, naturopaths, faith healers, acupuncturists, Big Pharma. Snake oil salesmen. The crime they are charged with is valuing personal financial gain over the act of healing.

The basic function of all master narratives is to uncomplicate. Like snake oil salesmen themselves, the guiding metaphors of our culture support certain belief systems and discourage others. That snake oil salesmen are liars is one such metaphor, even though in 2007, *Scientific American* found that Chinese snake oil does have curative properties. It can be used to relieve arthritis pain, improve cognitive function, reduce blood pressure and cholesterol, and alleviate symptoms of depression. Chinese laborers, who originally passed the palliative around to colleagues while building the transcontinental railroad, began to sell the stuff to passersby as the work they came to perform fell off and the railroad was completed. Snake oil became an industry all its own, a way of supporting the immigrant population convinced to leave their homes for the dangerous labor locals weren't sufficient enough in number to complete.

The Great Wall had convinced railway owners that the Chinese could meet the 4,400-worker labor shortfall they faced. In fact, the thousands of workers lured from Asia to perform labor-intensive and often life-threatening work took five years to complete the railway. (Thus the need for a soothing oil.) Of course, immigrant housing options in the late 1860s Wild West were nothing short of abysmal to start with. Once the tracks were laid, thousands of workers were put out of work, far from their homes, in a racially hostile environment.

It was the moment that made snake oil what it is (or is not) today. It's unclear if the laborers themselves began selling a locally produced but nearly ineffective version of the stuff to combat a poverty largely fueled by xenophobia and racism. Or if, having built up a following for their Chinese water snake oil–based curative, word simply spread beyond the original providers and substitutions were made to meet popular demand. Probably a combination of both, but what was sold after the railroad was completed was mostly a good story. Entire companies grew up around snake oil manufacturing, but without the Asian snakes necessary, they used a local alternative. Some used common ground snakes. Clark Stanley, who preferred to go be known as the Rattlesnake King, claimed the Hopi Indians taught him to use the deadly viper in his cure-all;[2] the Kickapoo Indian Medicine Company, too, claimed their snake oil followed Indigenous recipes.

That racial difference played a key role in snake oil's popularity among mostly white consumers is clear. But that the drive to expand the still-forming empire in any and all available directions—in this case, westward—belied some deep concerns about the newness of the American project is less so. Folks who'd just uprooted their lives, whether they came from already urbanized areas of the young USA or from elsewhere around the world, were being sold a story about the survival of ancient cultures and cures for human ailments that were thousands of years old. In many ways, the complicated falsehoods rumored to lie behind snake oil sales are themselves symptomatic of real fears endemic to American culture.

Despite widespread skepticism about the stuff, substances known as snake oil sold under that name for almost fifty years before the Pure Food and Drug Act came into effect in 1907, forcing consumables to be labeled with their actual ingredients.

♦ ♦ ♦

Some of my bottles of illusive liniments and curatives are branded with the staff of Asclepius. A single serpent winding around a knotted tree limb, it is the traditional symbol of the medical community. Asclepius was a physician in ancient Greece, later considered the god of medicine and healing. The snake—winding around the elderly physician's cane—represents eternal youth, what with the skin shedding and all. It is a symbol of regeneration.

Other bottles have two snakes, and a shorter cane topped with a pair of wings. This is actually the kerykeion of Hermes, also known as the caduceus of Mercury. It's the symbol of alchemists, occultists, and magicians: Hermes was the god of commerce and theft. This is a symbol of fast-talking trickery.

US history is riddled with confusion over the similarity of the images, a problem that some date back to the 1902 adoption of the caduceus as the symbol for the US Army Medical Corps. One presumes it is accidental when a government agency openly brands itself a sham, but who's to say? Real (by which I mean *traditional*) snake oils of my acquaintance, it should be noted, make use of neither symbol. They more frequently entwine a primary image—white man in a cowboy hat, stately white gentle-man—in two snakes, and do away with direct symbols of medicine and commerce entirely. Not to suggest this visual trope may not have been the source of confusion for the Army Medical Corps, however. Throw a couple snakes on something called medicine and sell it hard enough, and someone's likely to get confused about something.

Certainly, my snake oil saleslady didn't seem to care if she was ironically using the staff of Asclepius or unironically labeling her creations with the less-trustworthy caduceus. The ointments all look pseudo-official: they all give off the whiff of easily detectable deceit. After all, their creator put bath salts in a bottle labeled "smelling salts," and smelling salts in another titled "bath salts." And then, in a strange hat tip to the Pure Food and Drug Act—itself a response to complaints from snake oil consumers—properly labeled her own trickery.

Other slippages occur: Clark Stanley's Snake Oil Lini-ment turns out to be a *real snake oil*. Well: a *real* substance marketed under the term *snake oil*. In 1917 a shipment of the stuff was seized by border patrol agents. Scientists analyzed it and found it contained mineral oil, just as my *even faker* bottle does. The "real" snake oil liniment also contained a splash of red pepper, presumably to tingle the skin, and a single percentage of fatty oil. Not from snakes though—apparently from cattle, according to Lisa Hix in a 2011 Collectors Weekly article.[3] The final touch: trace amounts of turpentine or camphor weed, to make it smell medicinal.

Smell, it turns out, was crucial to the snake oil gambit. If you've ever spent a day installing a railroad and then sniffed yourself afterward, you can easily understand why.

Now imagine you're living in a frontier camp, and bathing hasn't caught on yet. Now pretend you're either European, Native American, or Chinese, and as invested as you and your fellow workers may be in getting this country up and running together, you're having a hard time trusting the unfamiliar. You need to find something you can all share.

♦ ♦ ♦

What we believe is not always true, what sells does not always work, and what is not available is not always inaccessible because it's ineffective. Sometimes a story is only accepted as truthful because it's been repeated so often. Even though you experience its falsities for yourself, you cling to the story. You believe it anyway.

When I was young, I would help my mom with the dishes and ask her about the fancy bottles lining the window above the sink. Their labels promised miracle cure-alls, decorated with long and elaborately coiled serpents and always, always, a white-haired, bearded man in a cowboy hat. These bottles had come from the reservation in South Dakota where she, a white person, and her doctor husband, another white person, had lived during the time I was born. And because that was far away, both psychically and physically, I was curious about these bottles, always. She would feed me answers, mixing up snake oil salesmen with medicine men, a pastiche of sepia-toned movie reels flitting through my head that included costumes such as railway engineer's caps, Mandarin headwear, ten-gallon hats, and feathered headdresses. Copious soap bubbles filled the sink as we talked, lending the air a gut punch of sudden cleanliness. Lineage and trade routes got confused.

When I would try to pinpoint the race of whoever had made or sold a miracle tonic, or any of its purported but potentially transplendent uses, my mother would grow annoyed. "It doesn't *matter*, Anne. They were all *fake*."

Her husband, my father, was a "real" doctor, sworn under the Hippocratic oath to share his personal wealth, heal his patients, refrain from seduction, and above all, cause no harm. He was also an abusive, philandering, racist alcoholic, and one of the most selfish men I have ever met. My mother remained wildly allegiant to him until he left her for the latest in a string of dalliances. Even at the age of six it was clear to me he was sleeping around, but the story that he was a healer, and kind, kept our family together despite mounting evidence for a quarter of a century.

When I remember those years of my life, I recall the smell of the air fresheners my father used to hang from the rearview mirror of his expensive car, their aggressive pungency demanding acceptance as natural. PINE™. STRAWBERRY™. FRESH BREEZE™.

It was unclear to me, growing up, exactly which fakery I was meant to be appalled by.

♦ ♦ ♦

One of the more disturbing undercurrents of the history of racial constructs is how visual differences became associated with differences of other types, each of which then fit easily into preordained strata of social acceptance. Secondary factors of racial difference were then easy enough to prove, in controlled environments. Presumptions about intellectual capacity, for example, could be easily tested with queries on issues of "common knowledge"—never mind that bodies of knowledge common to white American test administrators may be vastly different from those common to Chinese immigrants or Mexican Americans born south of the border who crossed into Texas in their own lifetimes.

The most striking of these secondary indicators of racial hierarchy, and perhaps the most persistent, was the belief that races were marked by smell. "Since the earliest contacts between Europeans and people of African descent, negative olfactory stereotypes have been wielded against those with dark skin," writes Michelle Ferranti in a 2011 issue of *Advertising & Society Quarterly*.[4] Thomas Jefferson contributed these thoughts in his 1784 *Notes on the State of Virginia*: "Besides those of color, figure, and hair, there are other physical distinctions proving a difference of race. They have less hair on the face and body. They secrete less by the kidnies, and more by the glands of the skin, which gives them a very strong and disagreeable odor."[5] J. H. Guenebault's 1837 translation of J. J. Virey's French tome, *Natural History of the Negro Race*, was another early example, claiming an odor existed that was unique to Black folk. In 1915, the French physiologist Dr. Bérillon claimed that odor formed the basis for racial animosity, in America and elsewhere, and it might never therefore be quelled.[6]

Ferranti points to a wave of incidents of "passing" after the American Revolution and before the construction of the transcontinental railway that had triggered some concern. Folks of African descent moving through primarily white cultures unmarked was upsetting to the self-defined, white-identifying society. Olfaction offered a curative: "If one could not visually detect someone's

African heritage," she writes, "they could at least smell it—or so it was claimed."

The claim, however, in matters of smell as in matters of snake oil sales, may be more abiding than the truth. In a 1995 cover story for the *New Republic*, Richard Klein writes of recent attempts to legislate the wearing of scents. "Perfume is threatening because it is so insinuating," he writes. An activist group had convinced the *New Yorker* to stop running perfume ads that contained scent strips, agreeing that "the reader had no way of escaping the smell throughout the issue, for perfume's very nature is to leak.... It is always unavoidable. Perfume never gives the smeller a chance."

It is partially due to its insinuating nature that smell remains the most elusive sense to vocabularize. Words for the act of experiencing smells are too few: I bet you can't name more than five. Now try to describe a smell. Frustrated? This is why we reach so often for the phrases "What's that smell?" and "Do you smell that?" when other senses allow us to maintain eloquence. Indeed, the metaphors for olfaction are more worn than others: old people's farts, something rotten, earthy. Each of these describe vast worlds of sensations that all reside on the socially-acceptable-to-downright-unpleasant continuum, but for the sake of accuracy I'd suggest they could stand a bit more parsing.

Kant would not have agreed. He felt that smell was the least philosophically significant of all the senses. It was too subjective, he thought, brought about too much immediate experience, didn't allow the intellectual distance for proper philosophical consideration. Yet one wonders if he was not pointing to a by-product of the limited language we use to describe smell, as opposed to anything intrinsic to smell itself.

The immediacy of odor has an upside and a downside, of course: The upside is that of all the senses, smell seems connected most intimately to our emotional core. A smart perfumer or florist or baker can wield that to easy advantage, and does: a smart real-estate agent will bake cookies in a house they wish to sell right before a viewing. The downside, however, is that without the vocabulary or intellectual objectivity with which to consider the matter, we could easily go on believing that rumors of foul odors justify xenophobia and racism, and never have a vocabulary to describe or uproot this process.

Smell doesn't need to be a powerful and mysterious force, in other words, guiding us toward and away from products and people with the help of our reptilian brains. We just let it.

♦ ♦ ♦

Here is what I understand: hidden under inestimable shrouds of trickery, somewhere, sometimes, can still lie a truth. Sometimes the fake can cure real ailments. Something with no power exerts it anyway. This is not a miracle, or mysticism; it is just nature. The master narrative is only one of several running narratives, and while you may wish to believe the one provable by sight, you may sometimes find yourself preferring, to your chagrin, the one deducible via scent. Or, perhaps, the reverse. They may be fungible. Sometimes the label you make up to store the fake cure accidently marks it as fake.

Sometimes, and this is true, I rub a bit of homemade

Clark Stanley's Snake Oil Liniment into a pulled muscle after a hard day. It smells tangy and clean but old, like wet rock. The label indicates that I should expect nothing from this liniment, or rather indicates both that I should and should not expect anything from it at the same time. But it is oily, it feels good, and I was told by my personal snake oil saleslady that it really works.

She was joking, but so far I have no reason to believe that she was wrong.

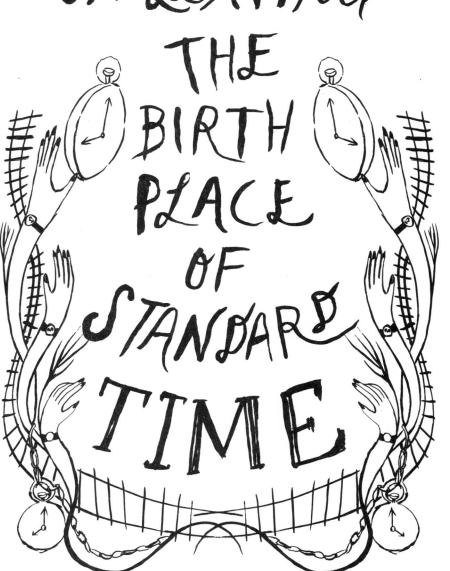

ON LEAVING THE BIRTHPLACE OF STANDARD TIME

I CAME TO CHICAGO at the tail end of 1993, a time and place that has been described as one of the most exciting in American music history. I went, at the time, to two or three shows a night, right up until I moved west six years later. When I left I wanted to go off-grid, to escape not the electrical grid but the urban one: the physical division of space along right angles, featuring sequentially ordered lot numbers, established in the spirit of a pervasive logic that allows you to look up from any outdoor location in the city and know exactly how many houses you are away from your own. It is a system that allows you to easily calculate how long it will take you to get to your house, or anywhere else, and the best means of crossing that terrain. And suddenly your life is efficient and predictable, and you feel accomplished for having figured out something so complex simply by looking at an address. Even if you have just stumbled out of a show at the Abbey Pub at 12:45 drunk as shit and are trying to get to the Empty Bottle to catch the headliners before they clamber offstage. A later analysis will reveal that each of the performers you traipsed around town to see that night had different careers by the next decade's end: one became an accountant, another joined the police force, two married and moved to a farm to raise twins.

You can calculate quite a bit about the future from any street corner in Chicago, but what you cannot predict is whether or not you will be happy there.

I found my first time away from the urban grid chaotic and distressing. Streets wandered aimlessly and adopted new names along the way. There were no means by which to tell how long travel might take within the city. Public transportation was spotty at best, and people were often late for appointments. I returned to the grid four years later. I had to get on with my life. I wasn't getting any younger.

▲ ▲ ▲

Chicago's grid system is more than a satisfying urban plan: it reflects the very origins of modern time, and the many efficiencies it birthed. Indeed, right at the intersection of Jackson and La Salle downtown, there's a plaque celebrating the adoption of standard time in 1883. The city had famously succumbed to a fire in 1871, in the days when there was no national system of time. Towns and cities with large railway stations relied on whatever time the massive, visible railway clock indicated; in the financial district of Chicago the most conspicuous clock was on the Chicago Board of Trade Building, so everyone used that. Clocks were all set to local noon, a fact that allowed for hundreds of local time zones. And this—this—is the thing: hundreds of local time zones made the creation of accurate train schedules kind of tricky.[1]

It's the oft-told tale of standard time: the railways developed, and then implemented, standard time in order to ease travel across great distances. And people, because they love being on time for things, responded to the notion of standardized time with great enthusiasm. Any close inspection reveals this to be a bold-faced lie, which we'll get back to in a moment, but pay close attention to the presumption embedded in this tale: that a single notion of time is universally desirable.

There was a time when I would have concurred that it was. Admittedly, it is hard to imagine a world that functions without being able to say, "Let's all meet up here at seven for a reading, and then I will read this very essay to you out loud, and it will take between seven and ten minutes, after which you can go home." Yet just because that is how the world functions now does not mean that other functioning worlds are not possible.

In fact, there was another means of going about daily life right up until 1883. At this time the Grand Pacific Hotel II stood at the corner of Jackson and LaSalle, a palazzo-style building constructed after the city was almost entirely destroyed in a fire. It was built to accommodate wealthy residents and well-off traveling businessmen, particularly those who did business across the street at the Board of Trade. In 1883 this hotel was where representatives from North American railroads decided to host the General Time Convention. At this meeting, the US was divided into five areas, each fifteen degrees farther from Greenwich, which translated into an hour's difference between each zone. (Alaska and Hawaii, now in separate time zones, were not yet a part of the Union.) The railway lines went about devising at this convention a means by which they would implement the change, and within a month it was done. Time had been standardized.

Note the key players in our story thus far: the robber barons that ran the railroads and high-stakes financial investors. Note, too, what goes unstated: that the standardization of time did not emerge from a popular uprising.

A little over a century later, in 1989, an astronomer, employee of what was then known as the US Army Laboratory Command, and time historian named Ian R. Bartky published an article called "The Adoption of Standard Time." In it he revealed that standard time was not initiated by the railways at all; in fact it was initiated by *astronomers*, who preferred to let the private interests of the railroads both do the dirty work of and take the blame for the fundamental shift in the way US residents arranged their days and interacted with one another that standardized time would require. Of course, this was calculated. People already hated the rich, who ran the railroads, but harbored few to no opinions about the scientists who looked at stars. Those scientists, however, needed a better way of communicating across great distances of land what was happening in the sky at the same exact time. Why not see if the railways could push forward this standard time thing, the astronomers figured, maybe get the job done? Pure science should not be sullied by such quibbles.

For it turns out that the standardization of time was enormously controversial. Bartky describes explosions and people shooting out the massive town clocks that the railways had installed—monuments to a hated temporal uniformity—in protest of the loss of individual determination over when things were going to happen.

What people were protesting the loss of, and how they got around *even on trains* before the introduction of standard time, was *talking to other people*. Business owners were angered by standard time because the railways holding a monopoly on time correctness meant no travelers had to step into stores to inquire after the local time. Unmarried young people were sad because eligible hotties passing through had no excuses to start conversation. And train porters, perhaps the most frustrated of all, saw full minutes shaved off of needed rest stops at several different points in their already long, overworked days.

Before standard time, in other words, when you went somewhere new, you had to get to know people to figure out how things worked there. The locals liked it. Travelers got by just fine. It seemed to work for everyone, in fact—except the astronomers, the railways, and the rich, who collectively found it easier to track planetary changes and fire people for being a few minutes late to work or for taking lunch breaks for too long.

The plaque itself, on the former site of the Grand Pacific Hotel II, commemorates Sunday, November 18, 1883, as the Day of Two Noons.[2] On that date, the text explains, astronomers at the Allegheny Observatory at the University of Pittsburgh transmitted a signal at noon on the ninetieth meridian, to which railroad clocks were reset. The plaque was presented to Continental Bank from the Midwest Railway Historical Society on November 18, 1971. See here that it simply restates in different language what I have already described: that astronomers gave the signal, the railways capitulated to it, and the banks celebrated it.

▲ ▲ ▲

A few years ago I accrued several debilitating diseases in a process some call falling out of time. I now function on crip time, which, to crips, means that we operate on a nonstandard schedule. We require more time to perform certain tasks than is usually allotted under the regimented, efficient system of standard time. The phrase is also used disparagingly. If you are invited to an accessible event, perhaps with ASL translators or requiring complicated maneuvers to allow wheelchairs entry, the able-bodied man sitting next to you may joke about crip time, by which he will mean that the event is starting later than he would like it to start.

I should mention that I was born on a reservation in South Dakota, where we had a similar concept called Indian time, although we described it otherwise. Indian time is the awareness that time—standard time in particular—is a construct of capitalism, and the doings of animals like people are not beholden to patterns of efficiency or imperialism. Nothing need proceed until the various spirits beckon them to convene, which is why I once spent four days waiting for a guy to teach CPR to my camp counselors, so I'm not saying that it doesn't take some getting used to. It is a term occasionally used pejoratively, yes, like crip time, but it is more often used with great affection. Indian time is differentiated, in South Dakota at least, from slow time and fast time because the latter refer to standard time zones that are arbitrarily adhered to in certain regions of the state based mostly on a whim. If one is late for a meeting, for example, one does not apologize by saying one is on Indian time; one says one has accidently set one's watch to slow time, to Mountain Standard instead of Central Standard. For if one is genuinely on Indian time, there is no reason to refer to other formulations of time, which do not matter. What matters is how your day is proceeding, what can fit into it, whether you have had enough rest.

This same concept is called something else in Latin America, and in the Styrian region of Austria, and outside of Tbilisi in the Republic of Georgia. From what I can gather, they don't bother calling it much of anything in the provinces of Cambodia because folks will just get to stuff when they're ready, if it really needs doing, and actually, why would you care what needs doing and what doesn't? Why don't you have a nap? It's hot out.

A similar principle is at work in crip time. When you get sick, it becomes clear real fast when something doesn't really need doing after all. I'm finding, more and more, that what I don't need to do, for example, is calculate from any street corner how to get to my next destination. In fact, I no longer wish to be destination driven at all. I am once again leaving the grid. While it's still technically true that I'm not getting any younger, I no longer care that I am getting older. In fact, a certain number of disease diagnoses in, I've learned to relish it.

To friends stuck on the grid for a while, or a lifetime, I leave you this thought: standard time, as natural as it now seems, has only defined certain humans for fewer than 150 years. It was implemented by scientists, bankers, and railway owners to ease their workloads and tax yours, in a decision that kept people from interacting with one another, from getting to know one another's individual needs and interests. Standard time need not last forever. Before its implementation, there were local times, and before that, maybe slightly different notions of time with separate sets of values distinguishing how individuals might prioritize their days. *Non*standard times still exist, everywhere, and serve to remind us that we matter as individuals, that our senses of well-being and personal abilities may not be best served by zones, alarms, deadlines, and grids.

"There is so much value," a reader named Asia wrote me

once over email from her home in Kampala, "in subverting standard time in big and small ways." In Uganda, she explained, certain celebrations, like weddings, parties, and graduations, start late on purpose. The things that really matter deserve your patience, the theory goes, and starting on time might signal to the audience that they do not truly deserve the experience of the event.

♦ ♦ ♦

Before the pandemic, the standardization of time felt wholly immutable. It was so deeply intertwined with how life worked, with the essence of how life *had* to work, that it was easy to mistake the coordinated doings of a few astronomers and railway owners 150 years ago for human nature.

The seemingly intrinsic logic of standard time was so tightly held by so many people that as the pandemic neared, it became increasingly easy to feel cast out of it, banished from the world of the living and consigned to another place, one that functioned suboptimally, where only losers reside. If you'd ever worked a night shift or been unable to shake jet lag after a trip, you were suddenly made aware of how significant standard time was to a sense of self-worth, an ability to connect with others, and one's movement through the world. If you worked from 10:00 p.m. to 4:00 a.m. and slept from 6:00 to 3:00, for example, you may have felt out of pace with society, an outsider or a criminal. Some feel dizzy when they drop out of time, others nauseous. It's amazing how quickly you can come to feel isolated if everyone is working while you sleep, or out playing. If you were the only person you knew on this schedule it did not feel good; if you found others who had also fallen out of time you could at least commiserate, and joke about the normies.

When the pandemic hit, we all fell into crip time. Events were canceled, rescheduled, and canceled again; strict deadlines lost rigidity, and people stopped wearing watches except to count steps or send emails. Industries reliant on speedy delivery—overnight shipping, journalism, financial services—developed lax approaches to customer service, although perhaps not always toward their own employees. Recall faded. Certain periods became truncated, while others expanded without limit: when meeting acquaintances you had not seen for years before the pandemic, it became common to trade stories of early pandemic survival but skip over whatever had led to the lack of communication in the years beforehand. Sending and responding to follow-up emails lost urgency, then currency. Making business inquiries on the weekend was suddenly forbidden. It was no longer necessary to apologize for missing an appointment. In fact, it quickly became unusual to do so, superfluous, because what excuse could you provide that was not already common experience?

Of course, I was used to it by then. Many of us who had fallen out of time long ago were used to it. We watched as all around us, masses of people were agog at the sudden crumbling of a beloved institution, standard time.

Yet no one lifted even the tiniest of fingers to try to save it.

CULTURAL IMPERATIVE

WHEN I BECAME pregnant I had recently gotten over cholera, a sudden-onset bacterial infection that causes intense cramping, extreme dehydration, and uncontrollable diarrhea. If you do not recover from it, you shit yourself to death. I had recovered from it, but suddenly felt one day a few weeks later as if I had not.

I'd gotten the cholera by drinking bad water from a pretty-looking mountain stream and, within hours, was either in bed or on the toilet, where I evacuated every last drop of water my body could take in through a variety of means. Food was immediately out of the question, and almost as quickly, drinking water became a waste of precious energy. I was wholly controlled by tiny agents in my belly that I could neither see nor touch, although their desires were made eminently clear in what I found myself doing at their behest: sleeping so as not to disturb them or emptying my bowels, over and over again, for their amusement. It nearly killed me.

I was barely recovered, still under a hundred pounds, when I felt a similar entity take over my body. I had had sex with a cis man, and shortly thereafter something shifted: how my inner resources were being allocated, what I was suddenly compelled to do. I felt controlled, invaded, run down, insignificant. It was horribly, awfully wrong. An internal force wanted to destroy me, still or again, and I knew I didn't have the strength to survive it.

"Something's wrong," I told my doctor when I could get in for an appointment. "I think I still have cholera."

She gave me a pregnancy test.

♦ ♦ ♦

For nearly two decades, I relied on the same party trick: presenting as a well-educated, upper-middle-class white woman of able body, I'd engage in polite but witty banter with fellow revelers until the topic of the Future would arise, and what each of us desired from it. Then came my time to shine! It made no difference in what terms the Future was being discussed—political, economic, domestic—because in every scenario women are consigned to limited roles, and my trick hinged on this fact. When it was my turn to speak (I liked to build tension by pausing to apply a fresh coat of lipstick) I would reject the options presented me. "I want to continue doing exactly what I am doing," I would say. I was unmarried, writing, and traveling extensively. "I am happy."

My declaration would first be met with silence (satisfied twenty- and thirtysomethings are apparently rare enough to stun). Then a well-intentioned and kindly voiced line of inquiry would emerge: "What about kids?"

"Kids?" I would say, gazing toward a far corner of the room, as if pondering the existence of the younger generation for the very first time. As if I hadn't been challenged on my disinterest in motherhood the night before, the week prior, the month previous, and for several consecutive years and now decades before that in a relentless social rejoinder to my consistent and apparently aggravating autonomy. "No," I'd say slowly, feigning consideration. "Not interested." And I wasn't.

Here, eyes would widen, and throats would be cleared. Glasses might crash to the floor, record needles might screech across LPs, a plane or two might fall from the sky. It seemed like it, anyway, for the gaiety would pause, and the mood in the room would shift. I'd failed to express a "healthy," "natural" desire to grow a baby in my tummy. Or however that works. What do I know? It wasn't really my thing. Worse: I had offered no apologies or explanations, and no defense of my position ever followed. For what else could I say besides no? For me, pregnancy was a full-body wrong. Even before this was proved to me I knew it in every cell. There was nothing to discuss.

At the party, a group of acquaintances, tongues loosened with liquor, would soon close in around me, a cacophony desperate to prove me wrong, inform me of my own naivete, accuse me of lying. My desire to make use of my body for creation but not for *procreation* was denounced in every way imaginable. The barrage of proclamations—on why I should want to become pregnant or did secretly want to become pregnant or would eventually want to become pregnant but did not yet realize it—could last late into the night. Some of these conversations trailed me for months or years and were revived at later parties, depending on whom I'd crossed paths with before and how they were feeling then about starting families.

Objections to my reproductive disinterest were telling in terms of volume and consistency, if not exactly logic. You see, the real trick wasn't the ease with which party-goers could be manipulated into haranguing me for an evening (this was too easy and, ultimately, very boring). The trick was on *me*, on *all people with uteruses*: the illusion of control we have over our own bodies and lives is less effective and more emaciated than we've been given to believe. My very bodily agency, it turned out, was considered up for grabs, even among close friends and trusted associates, in the most relaxed circumstances, on any night of the week.

▲ ▲ ▲

When the final decision in *Dobbs v. Jackson Women's Health Organization* was handed down—not too different from the draft opinion leaked months earlier, so no one could claim they didn't know what was coming, *Democrats*—I was in a fancy grocery store, too stunned to do anything but stare open-mouthed at my telephone while tears leaked down my face. I had woken up that morning a whole, regular, human person and now, with *Roe v. Wade* overturned and my constitutional right to terminate a pregnancy dissipated, I suddenly became something else. A vessel, but lesser: I'd been taking low-level chemotherapy drugs for nearly a decade and couldn't carry a pregnancy to term even if I'd wanted to, which of course I never did. A useless vessel, desiccated and abandoned. Valueless.

It took some time for me to compose myself, to recover from this sudden demotion from the ranks of humanity, and when I did, an older gentleman started a conversation with me. I'd spoken with him before and thought him kind: he asked me once how to cook rice, and what kind I thought his dog might like. Today he was agitated.

"They're not going to take much more of this, you know," he said, wagging his finger and speaking too loudly. "They've been getting beat up, and they're ready to fight back. Not just swinging punches either. Things will get violent." He shook slightly. With rage? Or disease? He was an older man. It could have been either.

In my lingering shock, and desperate for comfort, I flipped through the words I had just heard for some acknowledgment of this present moment, of this devastating day. Shouldn't he have said *women* at some point in that harangue? Or *you*? He hadn't. He wasn't expressing sympathy, it turns out. I clamped my mouth shut and cringed in anticipation of what he might say next.

"The Republicans have taken enough shit," he exclaimed.

The day prior, I might have said something like, "Yeah, man, imagine how people with uteruses feel!" Although obviously saying something like that wouldn't have made any sense twenty-four hours earlier. Which is not why I refrained from providing the snappy comeback. I didn't say anything that would have called attention to the complete solipsism of his worldview because he had just outed himself as someone who does not give a shit what my feelings are, or whether or not I have any. He had deemed me valueless.

These feelings, once I was able to articulate their many strands, were strong. For one, there was regret, for not having had many more abortions when I had the chance, and for not being able to go have one now, in my home state of New York, just to prove that I could. This rebellious, bitter swipe at authority would have not only meant making selfish use of a sought-after resource but also getting pregnant, so the urge soon passed. I also felt mournful that I hadn't devoted every single moment of my life to forestalling this eventuality, instead of just devoting a lot more of my time to it than most people did. Why did I sleep so much? Eat food so frequently? Watch movies? How could I not have understood how awful this would feel, to have a protected right stripped away, one that allowed me to move about the world with a greater degree of freedom, and with which people who were capable of giving birth might not always be forced to?

But mostly I thought—and I do now see how backward this is—of the next generation. Did I regret not having kids just so I could devote the rest of my days to educating them on the importance and means of reproductive justice? Not exactly. But sort of. I decided to go back into the classroom. Students have always come to me with their extracurricular difficulties, and it has often felt as if this were somehow impeding upon my ability to provide a real education. Suddenly I understood that extracurricular difficulties might allow for precisely the kind of education this moment required.

▲ ▲ ▲

Through years of cataloging the arguments that denounced my desire to remain childless, I watched certain patterns emerge. The most glaring of these posited that I had accrued some form of social debt by existing in the world that would eventually require repayment. The foundation of this stance wasn't that I would make a good mother (no one ever suggested that I would) or that an additional child would somehow be of benefit to the community (for babies, in my circle, are not so rare). Rather, it was that I might owe it—to society, to my family, to my ancestors, to "my people"—to reproduce.

Those of us who navigate the world as women often encounter hidden riders like these in the social contract, just as do trans and nonbinary people, and even cis men, whether these expectations get acknowledged or not. For gender is a form of debt bondage: we agree to perform the labor of femininity or masculinity or both or neither. In exchange, we are offered certain compensation, or no compensation. What forms those rewards take, the conditions under which they are granted or withheld, whether anyone truly owes anything to society in exchange for them, and toward what end the original agreement was negotiated and by whom are all worthy questions and deserving of an essay of their own. Here we will approach them only obliquely.

Let's focus now on how expectations of motherhood as the most appropriate form of productive contribution are often made explicit once someone read as feminine states a disinterest in bearing children. I'm certainly not the only cis woman who has faced the bizarre charge that I am wrong to want what I want—or, more exactly, that I am wrong to not want to do with my body what I don't want to do with it. That bodily desire can be labeled as wrong is a foundation of homophobia, racism, transphobia, ageism, and ableism as well as misogyny, but here we set the limits of our inquisition by the role I assumed at parties—that of a well-educated, upper-middle-class white woman with no visible physical malfunction; I cannot speak of any other experience.

There are, of course, plenty of others like me. The point of this essay is that an overeducated mind in a healthy-appearing, young, white body replete with feminine markers (in my case, more glitter and skirts than ample breasts or hips) and upper-middle-class bearing (*classy* glitter and *knee-length* skirts) is instilled with the message that she owes it to society to reproduce.[1] Women like me, we're told—by grade school teachers and college professors, church parishioners, friends in school, dinner party companions, or people we meet in the grocery store—are "well-bred" or "of good stock," and our obligation to procreate rests in part on the notion that we would raise the "right kind" of children. Judgments such as these stem from a particular mindset born of a particular context. In my case, perceived race, perceived education, and perceived class status mark me to some as the correct type of person to populate the planet. These exact phrases—*well-bred*, *good stock*, *right kind*, *populate*—have frequently been used to outline my responsibilities as an American woman. It is only now, in writing them down, that I can fully acknowledge them as massively problematic.

I should note that my disinterest in procreation is a form of privilege. Children are not necessary to my survival, and I could, during the years I might have born them, medically and legally ensure that I would not have them. I live in a time and place where, although it is an economic challenge to remain unmarried, it is not impossible, and as an independent woman, I have no partner's desires to consider as I pursue my own definition of family.

However, it must be stressed that pressures on me to bear children often appear to spring from a desire to shore up and extend the limits of this privilege to pass along to future generations imagined to emanate from my womb. This is a mildly flattering but deeply insidious form of elitism, class bias, and ableism, but most clearly I believe it to be rooted in—if not a fundamental mechanism of—white supremacy.

Let me state that more clearly: I think people have always urged me to have kids so there would be more white people in the world.

♦ ♦ ♦

It begins to seem possible to measure the precise value of my imaginary child, whose worth may well rival or best my own, inclusive of my social and cultural contributions. For when presented with an imagined future in which I must choose between bearing offspring and doing what I professed to enjoy—writing, creating art, and traveling—I have invariably been urged to choose the former, by both peers and figures of authority.

What makes this remarkable is that I am a reasonably well-respected (if modestly compensated) cultural producer, by which I mean that my livelihood and vocation are to create things that reflect the world as I see it, and I am allowed to do this because the work seems to hold value for people, who support me in creating it. Yet when the notion of children arises—I cannot call it a question because for me it is not one—my life's labor is relegated to prelude, the sideshow act before the main attraction, an imaginary child. The message seems to be that I've exhausted my individual worth on the countless zines, articles, magazines, and authored and edited books I've produced (seriously, I don't even know how many total literary projects I've completed), so now it's time to settle down and get serious.

Except that I have always been serious, have always known what I wanted, and was never swayed by anyone's suggestions regarding why I might be mistaken. Oh, I was still appalled by the arguments: the demand that I contribute to society invalidates what I may have already contributed to society, or whatever potential I felt at an early age I may have had to contribute to society eventually. That debt has been *paaaaiiiiiidddddd*, I thought, every time someone suggested to me anew that perhaps I might think about the next generation. (I've written several books for young people, and several more about my work with young people, and spent a full decade teaching undergraduates, so the idea that I haven't thought about the next generation is ludicrous.) But the mechanisms of debt are insidious: a month after paying off a credit card in full, you will always get another bill reflecting the interest accrued between the time your payment was sent and the moment it was received, plus the interest accrued on that total during the time you were sitting around thinking your account was clear. By then, you may owe a couple hundred dollars, basically for your own hubris in believing yourself to be debt free.

What I have come to understand is that, instilled in the agreement to perform womanhood, or perhaps all femininity, is an expected desire to be *re*productive, even if one has already staked a claim for oneself as *productive*. Creating things outside of the body may be seen as preparatory to creating something *inside* the body: that no matter what one has experienced in the public realm, a woman should eventually retreat to the private domain, for it is her rightful place. You have done a good many things in the world, and your work is strong, some partygoer or another always noted earnestly after I expressed my disinterest in having kids. But isn't it time to do something meaningful?

▲ ▲ ▲

The line between society and culture is often indistinct, but I am under no delusions that culture is anything more than the messy material by-product of people living in the world together and interacting socially—in fact, of society itself. So while culture may inspire many, often conflicting, definitions, the value granted cultural products in the United States is fairly straightforward. It is codified in a body of policy known as intellectual property, or IP, rights—laws that allow for economic, although not exclusively financial, gains and losses from the production of objects.

Consisting of trademark, patent, and copyright law, IP divides cultural production in the following manner: industrial language and methodologies are the domain of trademark law, scientific and design inventions are covered by patent law, and artistic creations are outlined in copyright law. Through a web of protections we consider rights, intellectual property is a primary conduit for the flow of capital around the world, the framework within which the trade in goods takes place. Yet what is protected under IP law is very specific: the tangible expression of an idea—the form—and not the idea itself. This is significant, and ultimately its ties to trade cannot be ignored: IP governs things and the ways they are made because objects can bear price tags. Indeed, the clearly stated goal of IP law, as legal scholar Madhavi Sunder writes, "is to promote the invention of more machines, from the Blackberry to the

203

iPod, and more intellectual products, from Mickey Mouse to R2D2."[2] The focus on the dissemination of tangible goods has a social and cultural effect, she argues in *From Goods to a Good Life*, her look at the interpersonal reverberations of IP policy.

Believe it or not, the human implications of object-based legislation are vast. Take for example the gulf between an idea and its expression—the period before which a concept is made tangible, before IP law can offer any protection. It's often called a pregnant space, or a space of gestation. (Creators awaiting copyright protection, inventors applying for patents, and businesspeople eligible for trademarks alike use terms like *birthing* and *baby* to describe pending projects.) This anthropomorphizing language matters. Particularly in IP law, where some potential forms of expression are wrangled into products and offered protection, while others are not. IP laws do not protect all potential expressions of ideas, in other words; they protect only the rights to certain ideas, when expressed in particular forms, and for the most part, when expressed by particular people. The equivalency between product creation and childbirth adopted in artistic, business, and scientific realms is no coincidence: IP laws and the manner in which they are applied tend to be quite gendered.

Copyrights, for example, cover creative expression within certain artistic mediums, the list of which reflects the historic roles of men as breadwinners and women as homemakers, as well as the cultural value of work created in the public versus the private sphere and for each implied audience, the general or the family. So while traditionally masculine forms of cultural production such as sculpture, filmmaking, and architecture are all copyright eligible, traditionally feminine forms of cultural production including food preparation, garment creation, and quilting (considered domestic labor because the products created are often intended for use in the home) are generally not. Patents, too, are offered to more masculine players than feminine players: in 2012, the National Bureau of Economic Research found only 7.5 percent of all patent holders in the US to be female, a figure that shrinks to 5.5 percent for holders of commercial patents.[3] This study has not yet been repeated, but more recent findings spark little hope for equity: in 2020, the World Intellectual Property Organization found that women were named in only 16.5 percent of international patents applications.[4] Not surprisingly, incidents of gender bias in patent-application and -approval processes are common, and some quite blatant— as in the long history of patent lawyers who would take ownership of women applicants' patents in lieu of fees. (Trademarks, which protect brand names and business practices, are gendered too—they cover products from which an overwhelmingly masculine group of CEOs profit—but, because they are more specialized, do not figure strongly in this discussion.)

The gendered presumptions on which IP laws rest, I contend, play a significant role in the sense that women may owe some kind of debt to society. My expressed determination not to reproduce—later made evident by a persistent lack of offspring—was met with a nearly despotic intolerance that did not waver with shifts in presiding politics or economics. I believe that the reason my prioritization of a productive role in culture and society over a reproductive one was so roundly rejected is related to why and how IP laws were gendered in the first place, and how they have evolved since. My suspicion is that intellectual property rights work not only descriptively, defining traditional roles for potential creators, but also prescriptively, consigning feminine players to one form of production and masculine players to another.

Echoing a concern of Sunder's, we might ask, how does a body of law that governs the production of things come to operate in relationships between humans? Of course capitalism, the economic system under which we operate, establishes a market to allow for survival through the trade of things. We—understandably—become emotionally invested in our abilities to retain goods available for trade or sale, since our survival would seem to depend on it. This ever-expanding market is where we buy in, literally, to the logic of legislation that governs the ownership of productive practices. Federal policy as individually held values system.

There is no question that humans retain certain beliefs even in the face of evidence that they do not hold true. Until quite recently, the productive drive was capitalism's most overbearing quality: the manufacture of clothing, food, and data in the United States has already far outpaced our desire for or ability to consume the same. Yet rarely have we ever questioned the need to produce more, or to be productive at all, and concerns that do arise about overproduction are quickly silenced by the accepted truth that economic security—for individuals and for the nation—relies on *producing things*. Stalled production under this values system is an indication of weakness, but failure to produce appears to be read as something far worse.

Since 2020, of course, we have been treated to a

different view on this same logic. Toilet paper, hydroxy-chloroquine, and baby formula were all at one point said to have been underproduced, manufacturers caught unawares by the consumer desires of the public under a pandemic and thus unprepared for increased demand; on the other hand, the supply chain was blamed for shipping delays of readily available volumes of auto parts, the paper necessary for print publications as well as books themselves, cosmetics, processed food. Shipping itself slowed, until two-day special delivery promises were regularly met days or weeks later. Stamp prices rose, for domestic mail and then, by an absurd amount, for international. Supply chain, supply chain, supply chain: the right amount of stuff exists in the world, or would exist in the world if certain players got their heads on straight. It's just getting it to the right place that gums up the works.

The peskiness of physicality! In a digital age we are urged to find bodies an inconvenience, to be annoyed that the right thing does not appear before us when we find we want it without having to move our own selves from place to place, or to have others move a desired thing to us. But the prizing of intellect, of concept, of desire, of demand serves also to deride human bodies and their many intriguing differences. Including the difference between who can and cannot become pregnant.

For those who can—or could conceivably—become pregnant, the failure to produce is where the space we have described as pregnant between an idea and its tangible expression becomes most significant. In IP terms, women who express no desire to birth children are unprotectable because there is no potential expression of this idea: nothing is produced. (Men who express no desire to raise children have many other sanctioned means of production to fall back on.) While capitalism might simply mark the absence with a big, fat zero, the values system incorporated by humans living under an ever-expanding market logic seems to identify it as a threat: a black hole of potential, horror vacui to be warded off at every turn. Under capitalism, then, when one expresses a desire not to produce—whether on the production line or in the birthing pool—one abdicates one's interest in protection. One proclaims oneself, it seems, valueless.

The implications of this extend well beyond my own diminished capacity to escape a cocktail party without catching a drink with my face: they have been seen in the regular repeal of federal abortion and reproductive-healthcare laws with glaring acuity. Politicians now seem to agree that women's reproductive value must be secured for the good of the entire nation. Forget the myth of the biological imperative. The imperative to bear children is cultural, and we have to stop kidding ourselves that it's anything else.

♦ ♦ ♦

The House Committee Reports on the Patent Act of 1952 claims "anything under the sun that is made by man" as its mandate of protection.[5] And from the precursors of modern patents in sixth-century Europe (*litterae patentes*, Latin for "open letters") up until quite recently, this description of the domain of patents—the driving force of the American economy—remained apt.

Originally official documents that granted privileges to their holders, early patents were especially useful to aid the exploration of foreign lands. As globalization scholar Vandana Shiva writes in her 2001 book *Protect or Plunder?: Understanding Intellectual Property Rights*, patents were originally used "for colonization and for establishing import monopolies."[6] The more modern notion of patents, as pertaining to the realm of idea-fostered objects and systems, emerged nearly a thousand years later in Renaissance Italy. At that time, the novelty of a device was figured regionally—in this case, in the Venetian domain—as well as based on the stature, or visibility, of the patent seeker within it. Uniqueness of a creation was less prized than its availability, so one did not need to invent a device to obtain an early patent; one needed only to manufacture a device that no one else within eyesight was already making.

Perhaps this seems counterintuitive. In our contemporary, globalized world, patent law is often used, alongside other IP and trade agreements, to dissuade local creation of a preexisting invention in what is usually called patent or IP infringement. Yet, in fact, the same distinction is at work, a legal framework that simply shifted allegiance as economic power centralized over time: as it became possible to track the proliferation of certain kinds of objects over greater and greater distances, patent laws increased the geographical boundaries within which they applied. Shiva suggests that the earlier mode encouraged technology transfer throughout the world, only to be replaced by a regime that prevents the global transfer of technology but is unsurprised when fluid definitions of creativity and technology are used to disadvantage certain actors. When patents came to the United States, for example, they were written to benefit US players. Under Connecticut law, *invention* was defined as "bringing in the supply of goods from foreign parts, that is not as yet of use among us."[7] Only later were import patents distinguished from patents of invention. Until then, finders were not only keepers, legally speaking. They were also *creators*.

The ambivalence in early IP law between what is created and what is found—the distinction between what is made versus what has merely been located and sited to a source that can be discounted in some manner (it is small, it is poor, it is in the Global South)—highlights interesting economic incentives hidden in patent law to encourage ignorance, travel, and self-promotion. Multiple patents were awarded around the world in the late 1700s, for example, for steamship creation, use, and travel ways, and a smart "inventor" could make a good go of business simply remaking the creations of others domestically. (The sheer number of patents assigned to preexisting inventions would testify to the likelihood that this happened quite frequently.) The ability to patent what has already been invented elsewhere offers financial benefits for a public life granted to masculine players but often denied to feminine ones. This is true in practice, certainly, if it is not inscribed directly into the law: women at the beginning of the 1800s stood a one-in-eight chance of dying in childbirth and bore an average of seven children in their lifetimes. Married women with the financial means to travel were surprisingly unlikely even to be able to get out of bed, much less locate a foreign invention to produce back home.

A quick accounting of the story of Samuel Slater can illuminate the ripple effect of gender biases in patenting. Born and apprenticed to a cotton miller in England, Slater departed for New York in 1789 after committing locally patented cotton-spinning secrets to memory with the intention of selling them in the States. For his plundering he was named the Father of the Industrial Revolution by Andrew Jackson, although locals in his hometown referred to him as Slater the Traitor. It's unclear what he was called by the laborers who worked in the factories he is said to have revolutionized because as female members of the underclass and/or recent immigrants, their genders, races, and class deemed their specific contributions unworthy of public note. (This, of course, equally applied to their innovations to his designs and explains their absence from his patent applications, although they are likely to have offered improvements fairly consistently in the course of their work.) Indeed, Slater may have been known as the Father of the American Factory System, but what he really innovated—through theft—is textile manufacturing. Today, around one in seven women who work outside the home labors in some aspect of the textile industry, a workforce that on average brings in far less than half the amount of money it takes to survive in the regions of the world in which they work. Slater can't be held exclusively responsible, of course, but his legacy includes a significant contribution to the global gender wage gap.

Due to the manner in which they foster and restrict global trade—indeed, how they limit those who might profit—patents, even more than other forms of IP (including copyrights, which have been around exactly as long), form the backbone of American-style capitalism. Thus our political economy rests on gendered constructs—and it always has. Yet since the first US patent was awarded in 1790 for making potash, a salt used in both soaps and artillery, patent protection has been described as an unbiased stimulator of creativity, a protective measure for the makers of products that offers exclusive rights to profit from patented goods.

Patents are uniquely aimed to incentivize cultural products, elements of processes, or technological solutions in "Science and useful Arts," as the US Constitution explains. They are guaranteed only on successful application and cover a significantly shorter period than copyrights (twenty years from date of application, in most cases). There are three main types of patents: utility patents, which apply to processes, machines, products, material, or a significant improvement to previous versions of any of these; design patents, which cover the ornamentation or decoration of a manufactured good; and plant patents, which are awarded to those who invent or discover a unique or innovative kind of plant.

Theoretically, of course, exclusive rights to profit may spur makers toward innovations—or theft—but there's very little evidence to show that economic gain truly stimulates the creative process. And there's none to show that women and other marginalized folks have been offered similar incentives to create, however much they persist in doing so in the absence of the right to profit. In fact, the notion of patents as creativity stimulators is fairly quickly revealed to rely on an unproven logic that ignores inherent masculine privilege and confuses legal rights, financial gain, and free expression to create the myth of US ingenuity and entrepreneurship. More than anything else, patenting seems to uphold the myth that we Americans pull ourselves up by our bootstraps (#US 216544, patented by Henry M. Weaver of Mansfield, Ohio, in 1879).

Yet who made that boot, and who waxes those straps?

What patenting deliberately fails to acknowledge are the communities and contexts that often lead to what we call invention and discovery. Sunder rightly notes that colonialism, gender bias, and racial and economic stereotypes tend to credit innovation to the most visible, not the most innovative, who are also often the most poor. One of the noted areas in which the poor—farmers, in the cases she describes, often in developing nations—have seen contributions overlooked is in agriculture and medicine. Recently, patents for herbs long known to promote certain healing effects in India, for example, have been awarded to US companies. It's a situation that started in 1931 with the first plant patent, which covered distinct varieties of asexually produced vegetation. It was the first time that life-forms became subject to intellectual property claims, but it was not the last.

In 1988, a sea change: the first patent was awarded for the ownership of and rights to profit from a living mammal. #US 4736866 was granted to Philip Leder and Timothy A. Stewart of Harvard University for the creation of the OncoMouse™, a mouse they'd bred for cancer research. No longer were patents covering the vast domain of "anything under the sun that is made by man." For the rodent was at least partially made by an impregnated female mouse, who went unnamed in Leder and Stewart's application.

♦ ♦ ♦

Whether to mice or men, offspring-producing female mammals ceded then their formerly exclusive domain, the creation of new mammalian life-forms. The changes to patenting were significant, but also not, for the new patent revived earlier, ambivalent definitions of certain key terms: an invention could be found; a novelty could be elsewhere common. The new domain of patent ownership also revived an even older notion of patents from the sixth century, when they were intended to aid exploration and colonization. Is it not colonizing to invent new forms of mice over which you retain a great degree of control? So the patenting of mammalian life in 1988 didn't happen suddenly, although it did suddenly lay bare the gendered intentions of IP policy. Although even that had a precursor, a quarter century earlier.

Up until the mid-1960s, most things under the sun that were made by women weren't truly owned by anyone at all. The forms of cultural production to which women were often consigned were not considered authored in the contemporary sense and were therefore not eligible for IP protection. Dinner just appeared on the table, and clothes emerged from closets. Of course, women were actively dissuaded from participating in patent-heavy STEM fields, partially because babies. And babies didn't require IP registration; they were simply birthed. Some of them grew into *men*, who could be said to be made by pregnancy, specifically, or maternity, more generally. Yet the rights to profit from their output? Somehow retained by the men themselves.

In 1964, a patent (#US 1970000062143) was awarded to William Wright and Ralph Meyerdirk for the first articulated-arm scanner, also known as the sonogram machine. Heralded as a means by which pregnant women could bond with unborn fetuses, ultrasound technology rose to popularity quickly. Sonograms made the previously hidden mysteries of life visible, although not exclusively to the women it was presumed weren't already bonding with the fetuses growing inside them. At this time, men—husbands, older brothers, male doctors, interns, medical technicians—were granted access to this previously unseen provenance too. (Given the frequency with which they were denied entry to hospitals in general, I would be surprised if women and nonbinary partners of pregnant people were granted similar viewing rights.) This shift had a cultural parallel: in the 1950s, it had been common to announce, "We're having a baby!" while the same sentiment two decades later might be expressed with the biologically less likely "We're pregnant!"

IP rights to an unborn creation may not have changed yet—they would, however, and soon—but the cultural sense of ownership over a pregnancy certainly did. Sex education adopted a spiritual tone, situating intercourse as the scientific foundation of life itself; the interiors of women's bodies were photographed, stripped of actual women, who became mere background to fetuses, the nonconsenting models on the covers of news magazines. The ownership of pregnancy, in other words, became cultural through the wonders of ultrasound technology.

If we accept that sonograms provide pregnant folks the opportunity to increase their emotional attachment to growing fetuses—and I'm not convinced that we should, although my disinterest in participating in any aspect of the process may be coming into play here—we can expect that sonograms would elicit a similar response in the men partners of pregnant people. Or, perhaps, in men in general. After all, recent studies indicate that social media—which facilitates interaction between physically disconnected social actors—does provide many of the same effects as in-person interaction. If the argument runs, in other words, that a person will bond more quickly with a fetus they can view inside their own body, it stands to reason that a person will bond more quickly with a fetus they can view inside the body of another.

The exact psychology at work, however, may matter less than the political impact of a technology that allowed men unhindered visual access to the interior of women's bodies. In 1988, twenty-four years after the patenting of the ultrasound machine allowed a broad swath of people greater insight into the mechanics of pregnancy, the first patent was granted that guaranteed ownership of mammalian life. Note that twenty-five is the exact minimum age required for election to Congress, which in 1988 was 95 percent male. So the men who voted on whether other men should have the legal right to own and profit from the creation of mammalian life-forms were the first generation of men to grow up—literally, not metaphorically—under the watchful eyes of their fathers *since conception*, all thanks to a device from which other men profited.

Masculine ownership of the means of *re*production, I'd like to suggest, was gradually normalized throughout the second half of the twentieth century. First in the early 1960s through the sonogram machine, and then as images of what the machine allows us to see were circulated throughout popular culture. In some cases, these were printed and stapled to wooden struts, deployed to convince pregnant people not to abort. This shift in control over reproduction was furthered in the late 1980s with the patenting (and trademarking) of the OncoMouse™.

Perhaps before 1988 there existed such a thing as a biological imperative, a drive described as natural that some suggest lies at the base of a desire to bear children; it seems possible that maternity may have lost some of the purely biological veneer since. It could be (and has frequently been) argued that the planet no longer requires or even supports an expansion of humankind, and that the biological imperative, if it did ever exist, is no longer necessary, sustainable, or ethical. It may only be left over, a relic of life before technology. The urge toward pregnancy is now largely cultural.

▲ ▲ ▲

When I needed to exercise my then constitutionally protected right to abortion, I was living in the Midwest, working at a leftist magazine during the day and a comedy newspaper at night, and on the weekends I self-published a fanzine. It was the easiest thing in the world to tell my coworkers, "Oh, I'm sorry I cannot go to work on such and such day because I need to have an abortion." I found my provider by flipping open the pages of the magazine I worked at and reading a column by a local doctor who had recently begun wearing a bulletproof vest to work. I called her from the magazine's office and had an initial appointment as soon as they could fit me in.

Wisconsin, at the time, was already chipping away at the protections offered in *Roe*. There were sixteen clinics when I moved there after college in 1993, and by 2014 there would be only four. State law in 1994 dictated that I attend a counseling session before my procedure, speak to a healthcare provider, and receive a packet of "information." These were images that might dissuade me from having an abortion, and perhaps a brochure or two about adoption or fetal heartbeats, decorated with even more images. It was preposterous, and everyone I spoke to that day knew it. Somehow, my counselor managed both to hear my description of my physical state as "wrong," "bad," and "a disaster," and to hand me a packet filled with images curated to convince me that this wrong bad disaster was natural, joyful, and God's will—all without judgment. Neither of me nor, more distressingly, of the packet of propaganda she handed over. She also managed to convey to me that, although I clearly understood what my body needed, the law demanded I wait twenty-four hours before making the appointment for the procedure.

Inside the packet were pictures of fetuses at various stages of development—all possible though Wright and Meyerdirk's invention—as well as photographs taken outside the pregnant body, of fetuses in varying states of dismemberment and/or decay. It will not surprise readers of this book that none of this dissuaded me in any way from the medical decision I was making about my own body, nor will it surprise you to learn that I became so enchanted with this packet that I went on to write my master's degree thesis on abortion-rights imagery in popular culture (where I would come to learn that such images were often of stillbirths or other, more complicated medical procedures, not the voluntary D&C I was then hoping to undergo).

My emotional terrain over the course of that twenty-four-hour waiting period was rocky. Let me be clear: no part of me doubted that abortion was the correct biological, emotional, physical, economic, professional, and spiritual decision for me. It fit, yes, into my own life and career plan at the time, but within a few years it would also become obvious that it was the best medical decision I could have made under any circumstances. Yet as horrible as I felt playing host to an unwelcome invader, I also felt bad for being such a shitty hostess.

What the images meant to do was horrify me with the impact of the medical procedure on an identifiable humanoid form. (I was clearly supposed to bond with the photographic subjects.) On this front the packet failed. But what the existence of the packet made clear even in the mid-1990s was that a large and politically influential body, a growing force in culture, was becoming more insistent in its demands that I abandon the creative life for a procreative one, give up being productive and become, finally and exclusively, reproductive.

The cultural imperative wouldn't relent, I saw then; it would only grow, deepen, and become more insidious. There was no part of me that could conform to it, then or ever. And that—guess what?—doesn't feel good. To enter a situation by choice that will make a lot of people angry with you for the rest of your life is not a decision to be undertaken lightly.

♦ ♦ ♦

These days at parties, I'm more likely to be asked how many kids I have than when I am going to have them, but my answer hasn't much changed. Sometimes I offer a spluttering recitation of a full life and active career, and other times I state dully, "I've written, like, twelve books." I admit I have occasionally mentioned my cats. Whatever my response, I'm still expected to defend my childlessness, my selfishness, confronted about my apparent disinterest in honoring my parents, or just plain asked what is wrong with me. (While I do have several invisible chronic illnesses, not a single one of them played into my decision to remain childless, so they do not enter this conversation.)

Neither does the measure of my cultural production mitigate the implicit accusations, the sense (we all feel it) that I have erred. Still, somewhat regularly, I am called upon to explain my aberrational nature, of being a woman apparently capable of having children who won't. It's not only straight white cis men demanding justification. It's my South Asian immigrant former neighbors, the university-educated attendees of my visiting lectures, new acquaintances, book-event visitors, fellow dinner companions, my own students. Inquisitors may express considerable interest or even investment in my work but remain reasonably sure that my output is not enough.

In such conversations, I feel it most clearly: being a woman who is a cultural producer is an insufficient fulfillment of my obligation. I will not be valued, it seems, until I become a *reproducer*. I suspect this may be true as well for women physically incapable of pregnancy, may contribute to the sense women gain as they age past childbearing years that they are no longer of value to the world.

This may be due, in a very basic way, to the ways in which intellectual property rights laws have forced us to value notions of production and various potential producers. IP laws outline a particular course of roles for masculine players and another for feminine players and then police them, at least partially, through the assignment of copyrights and patents. "We must understand intellectual property as social and cultural policy," Sunder rightly contends of the laws that govern who we value as productive and who as reproductive.[8] For the valuative system implemented in IP law does seem to show up again in individual relationships—even between random partygoers, when collectively imagining their futures.

My concern, and my frustration, is that this contributes to a sense that pregnancy for whoever can manage it is obligatory, although cast as biological desire. If, as many have contended throughout the history of IP law, the entirety of intellectual property rights were established as a counterweight to the ability to birth babies, those who physically can must reproduce as long as cis men keep producing. The logic of one proves the logic of the other. It starts to seem like a sad race to make more stuff and more people to make use of it, not out of desire for bounty or joy for the future, but because we are told we must, in a logic so deeply instilled we write it all off as natural.

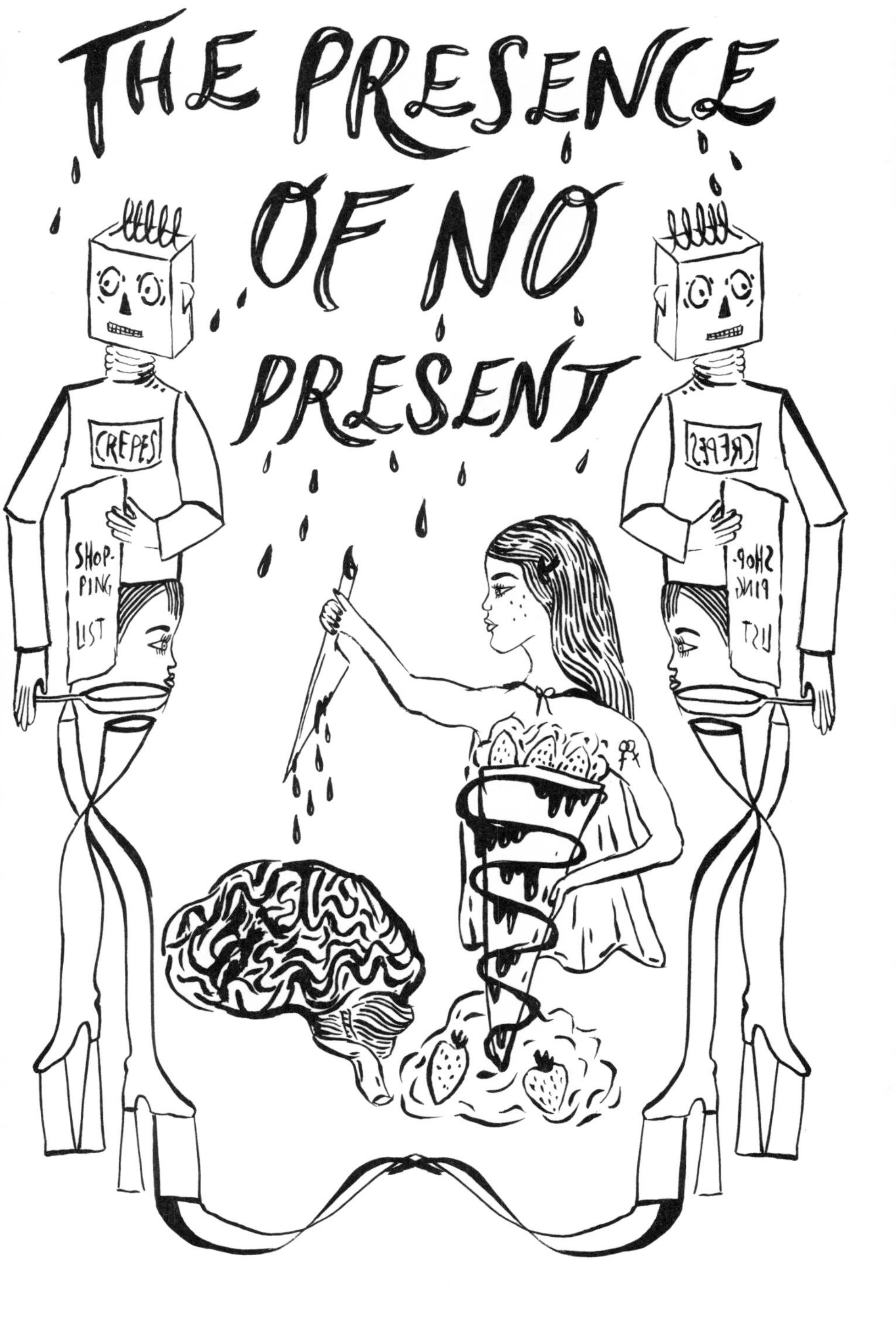
THE PRESENCE OF NO PRESENT
CREPES
SHOP-PING LIST

AUTOCORRECT FUNCTIONS IN voice-to-text modes across all personal digital communication platforms that I use change *queer crip* to *queer crop*, or a similar mistranslation. *Clean crepe* has also appeared, and once, *queen creep*. My physical impairments, the results of any of a variety of chronic illnesses I navigate daily, make it painful to change, once, again, and then a third time, which is about the number of manual corrections I must perform in order to make it clear to the machine what I intend it to automatically transcribe.

This is not so unusual. It is similarly difficult to make myself clear in direct conversation with other people: "Not crit, *crip*," I clarified once, speaking to a young man at a bonfire. "As in *crippled*? The reclamation of an offensive slang term by the folks it is generally used against in an effort to own its power? Also in recognition of it being a badass word thanks to media depictions of gang culture? Were you not alive in the nineties?"

Indeed, the young man I was speaking to was born in the 1990s. His earliest memory of the culture of that time period occurred over a decade later, when a grade school pal played him Nirvana for the first time. He told me he loved the oldies.

This is less an essay about aging, however, than it is about the limitations of perception. I lived, for example, with a shifting repertoire of physical impairments for a little over a year and a half before I became accustomed to classifying them as disabilities. Still, the difficulties I experience physically navigating the world pale in comparison to those I faced making others initially understand that I suddenly required particular consideration regarding food, travel, and endurance activities like walking more than a block. It took, I mean to say, over eighteen months for me to recognize that others also deal with such circumstances—all the time—and that in fact there is a long and amazing history of disability-rights activists, organizers, and scholars who have worked extremely hard to secure legal recognition of their particular needs, not only for themselves but for others, and to overcome barriers far more pronounced than my own in an effort to make my life easier, should I find myself relying on their foresight. I am, let me be clear, neither stupid nor ignorant of political struggles in history; indeed, I have studied radical uprisings closely. I teach critical art theory around what a cultural reliance on visuality means for those with visual impairments. I have worked closely with disability-rights activists and advocates for healthcare reform on intersectional projects. Upon reflection, then, it strikes me as extremely strange that for eighteen months, neither I nor anyone I knew labeled my daily struggles "disabilities."

I admit I became fascinated, then, that my curiosity about the history of disability rights was spurred only when I needed to understand how folks in the past had dealt with the workplace discrimination, lack of medical support, and pervasive, isolating ableism that I was now navigating as a matter of course but felt so comfortable in less than two years before. Yet when I wanted to find out more, there were shockingly few accessible resources to turn to.

What I want to point out is that the historical erasure of crips, as reflected in the recent dormancy of that word itself, contributed directly to my inability to describe my lived experience to others. In fact, the communication struggle became at that time another barrier, an additional impairment to my engagement with society. We might begin to think about the historical erasure of crips as a *cause* of disability.

▲ ▲ ▲

Consider the function of language for a moment. It is, in theory, my field as a writer. I don't like to brag, but I know a lot of words. Like everyone else, I use them to make sense of the world. Additionally, my vocation is stringing them together to form communicable ideas. You may be surprised to read that I am doing this, even now.

The linguist Roman Jakobson described in 1960 six potential functions of language: the referential, the poetic, the emotive, the conative, the phatic, and the metalingual—of which this paragraph is an example, as we are both using language and describing the function of language. Distill these strains even further and we can see that language exists so that engaged parties can share information and ideas about one another and/or the world.

The use of language to describe oneself has a long history, of course—Plato wrote about it in his Allegory of the Cave around 380 BC. More recently the use of self-referential language has become a focus of public concern, as in the decrying of identity politics, qualms with demographic marketing, or providing pronouns. The entire project of branding, too, is all about finding the right word and associated image to identify with to allow oneself to be categorized, and for this reason alone I am often slow to participate in choosing self-descriptors. When I do adopt a defined term to explain myself or my desires, I do so carefully.

That being said, I have identified as queer since I first heard the word. The sonance of it somehow transmitted perfectly my ambivalence toward what everybody else seemed to want that failed to intrigue me: queer in the anti-capitalist sense. The structures set up to ease hetero-sexual coupling at every stage of our economy, society, and culture don't do it for me. Neither does the supposed goal of birthing children, although I tend to enjoy the young that others have birthed when I meet them. The word *queer*, as I use it, signals my rejection of the idea that identifying as a woman is a tacit agreement that I will stick to certain established pathways, whether emotional, professional, sexual, or financial. Queerness, to me, is a refusal to situate myself as a feminized subject of capi-talism. Such a stance demands skepticism toward the seductive lifestyle brands that so often cheerlead the mile markers along established life pathways: I have never purchased, for example, a yogurt or item of clothing based on a supposed but well-ballyhooed affinity for the LGBTQ+ community. To me, *queer* is shorthand for "stop telling me what I want and how to acquire it." That there is also enor-mous pleasure in physically desiring a wide range of body types and gender identities and to be found within a pleth-ora of scenarios is, for the purpose of this essay, none of your fucking business.

Crip could function similarly. (For a lot of people, it does.) Those established pathways—from high school to college, or dating to babies—have fairly deep grooves. The built environments created to guide a so-called normal human body along its course are unevenly constructed. Sometimes they crumble inconveniently and uninterestingly. They do not account for all types and therefore aren't always accessible. They rarely get me anywhere I want to go. *Crip* could mean "let's cut to the chase and both admit you know nothing about my bodily needs."

Yet I admit that when I first heard the word *crip*, way way back in the 1990s, I did not similarly identify with it. I could not identify with it. That took the accrual of several debilitating diseases, and then, interestingly, another eighteen months.

It is fascinating, isn't it, that one might know the precise name for something but refuse to apply it to oneself? Racists, I think, do this: see that a word exists to differentiate those who believe a system of oppression can be justified on the unproven grounds of racial difference, but fail to apply it to themselves. Perhaps they feel the term *racist* is pejorative—some do—and therefore can't accept it as a self-description because their beliefs were come to out of love or a misapplied logic.

Maybe, partially, this was my problem too: I couldn't be a crip because crips were . . . what, I don't know. Other. Necessarily unknowable to anyone who was given to believe that they were normal. But also, it is a word, and not one commonly used in the midwestern cities I grew up in—or, frankly, the northeastern agricultural community I live in now. If language exists so that people can share information and ideas about one another and the world, it fails when vocabulary is unshared. The word *crip* holds no meaning for too many people. It is a signifier lost, a sign that points nowhere. I couldn't be a crip growing up not only because my body appeared to function in a normative way, but also because no one would know what it meant.

One way to elucidate the failure of a dominant system is through language: crafting vocabulary to identify the constituent elements of a shoddy structure, articulating points of weakness or inflexibility. Indeed it is, as we have established, a function of language to communicate that which may otherwise not be evident immediately. For language to function as communication, all parties must share vocabulary, must be open to new words and meanings, and must generate the patience required to adapt to them. The parties must revive those terms that have fallen into disuse or otherwise ensure that the concepts they represent are not ignored or abandoned. The word *crip* proves this is not assured; the word *crip* proves that, in fact, the disinterest in certain forms of difference is very resilient indeed.

The inability to properly utilize words: we call people who suffer this condition illiterate, ignorant, or stupid. Perhaps, if we are being kind, aphasic, dyslexic, or still learning. I spent twelve months responding to my disability by taking medications that are also used to treat certain forms of cancer. These medications cause what is referred to in medical communities as brain fog, and during this time I often struggled to remember certain common words. Rather, I am *told* I struggled to remember them; in truth I formed no memories during this time, a year during which anything could have happened. Perhaps it is an explanation for my inability to identify myself in language that was already familiar to me: my internal vocabulary system was malfunctioning.

Yet I suspect that a larger malfunction was taking place, too, and is still ongoing: an erasure of queer disability narratives that is broader than, although indicated by, the loss of meaning of the single, infrequently recognized term *crip*.

▲ ▲ ▲

Someone sent me a robot, the marketing materials for which promise to make my life easier, although in reality it just tries to get me to order things from Amazon Prime. Occasionally it plays me music at my request, as long as the artist I want to hear does not have a name that is similar to any other word, phrase, or concept in the English language. Ostensibly to soothe my overly taxed memory, but likely to make it that much easier to order from Amazon Prime, this robot automatically culls shopping lists based on what it believes I want but do not already own, which it compiles from what it believes I have said to it. This shopping list currently reads:

— calendar
— tips
— thesaurus
— cinnamon for permeability
— tips

I am unsure what will happen when it mishears something normal I say as, "Go ahead and buy all that shit off of Amazon Prime, but that's a very specific kind of cinnamon I like so don't eff it up." Obviously it will do this, though, because this is the future, and the future is a freaking mess.

Allow me to illustrate. I wanted to know something completely normal, something that probably every human alive has ever wanted to know, and I thought to ask this robot, even though this is the worst robot I have ever experienced in reality or movies or my imagination, counting even robots designed by evil scientists to murder people. Here is an exact transcript of that conversation:

Alexa, does it hurt to get stabbed in the brain?
Sorry, I couldn't find the answer to the question I heard.

Alexa, how much does it hurt when you stab someone in the brain?
Sorry, I couldn't find the answer to the question I heard.

Alexa, what do you know about brain stabbing?
Sorry, I couldn't find the answer to the question I heard.

The machine that has been designed to live in my house and make my life easier by ordering me things off of Amazon Prime is totally useless.

Alexa, you are completely useless.
Sorry, thanks for the feedback.

But the problem that the very existence of this robot points to is real. Eventually, I will need to find some way to deal with the fact that my right arm is losing function, and that this does, in fact, make shopping difficult. I had high hopes. The week the robot arrived, I had visited a hematologist to find out more about a new genetic disorder that I just found out that I have and that I suspect, based on my research, could be causing my meds to fail. But the hematologist didn't know anything about it, so he called his boss, who also didn't know anything about it, and then he called *that* guy's boss, who *also* didn't know anything about it. In the end, the first guy, the hematologist, told me that I was very smart, and likely correct, but that he would not be able to help me in any way. All he could do (and, thankfully, did) was make sure I was not charged for the unhelpful visit. As I left his office, he called me back again to ask me to promise to contact him once I figured out whether or not my genetic mutation was causing my medications to fail because he thought it would make a very good subject for a research paper. Let me repeat that for you: my fucking blood specialist asked me to act as his goddamn unpaid fucking medical consultant in lieu of helping me get treated.

You can see why, as a person with a rotating spate of physical impairments who can't seem to get them properly medicated but is asked, nonetheless, to donate medical findings to those who fail to provide any assistance whatsoever, a robot that lives in my house and makes my life easier *in any way* might be appealing, *even if that way is to perform the sole function of shopping from a single online store that I also happen to hate.*

> Alexa, what is the *most* painful place in the body to get stabbed?
> *I've added "body" to your shopping list. Is that correct?*

> Jesus. Fine. Alexa, I've had a shitty day and would love to hear some oldies. Play me some Prince.
> *I've added "tips" to your shopping list. Is that correct?*

In *Feminist, Queer, Crip*, Alison Kafer takes issue with Marge Piercy's erasure of people with disabilities from her feminist sci-fi utopia *Woman on the Edge of Time*. In the novel, no characters exhibit any evident impairments: people with disabilities have been erased. Without addressing disability, or presenting people with disabilities as deserving of inclusion in utopia, Kafer explains, Piercy performs a particular kind of violence that she refers to as "the future of no future."[1]

The tiny robot that lives in my house and tries to get me to order stuff off of Amazon Prime is an emissary from this future, creating what we might call, building on Kafer's notion, the presence of no present.

Alexa, what do you know about people with disabilities?
Sorry, I couldn't find the answer to the question I heard.

Alexa, do you know what a crip is?
A crop, sometimes called a riding crop or hunting crop, is a short type of whip without a lash, used in horseback riding, part of the family of tools known as horse whips.

No. Alexa, do you know what *crip* is?
Create.

That's not even an answer. Alexa, do you know what *crip* is?
The Committee for the Re-election of the President, abbreviated CRP, but often mocked by the acronym CREEP, was a fundraising organization of United States president Richard Nixon's administration.

Alexa, goddammit. Do you know what *crrriiipppp* is?
Sorry, I couldn't find the answer to the question I heard.

Okay, Alexa. Do you acknowledge that people with disabilities exist in the world?
I don't have an opinion on that.

It's a record-scratching moment deserving of some consideration. Clearly, a programmer flagged something in this generic query about the existence of people with disabilities as potentially controversial, and slotted in a standardized palliative, the soothing response provided whenever issues of great trauma arise in Alexa's presence. Questions I asked the robot about religion, the death penalty, and abortion elicited similar responses, although these were not questions about whether or not religion, the death penalty, and abortion *exist*, which raises alarm. For there is little so dystopic as a future that does not recognize you, that finds even mention of your existence controversial.

♦ ♦ ♦

During my eighteen months as an unidentified queer crip, I pitched, on four occasions, stories to editors who were initially delighted by the idea of publishing a lighthearted but thoughtful take on chronic illness and disability. Once the stories were submitted, however, they were never quite lighthearted enough, or they were too lighthearted, or otherwise just wrong. Unprintable, is the point.

On one occasion, I was told I'd "missed my opportunity" to make an essay on autoimmune disorders interesting to readers when I turned it in pegged to a news hook that was then twelve hours old. By some accounts, the number of estimated autoimmune disorder sufferers in the US approaches fifty million, which most editors would consider a large potential readership, although it is true that, under the prevailing logic of the twenty-four-hour hot-take news cycle, a story that comes in twelve hours late may indeed have missed its mark. Yet to an under-informed but afflicted 16 percent of the population, all takes are hot. (This was well before the pandemic made clear that the specific needs and interests of people with autoimmune disorders and other so-called comorbidities were entirely separate from, if not antithetical to, the news-reading public.)

After I turned in a different piece, a second editor—able-bodied, natch—explained to me what a proper disability narrative included and why my essay failed to conform to it. She wanted me to present a problem in the first hundred words that could be tidily overcome after twenty-five hundred of them, and then overcome it. Of course, such a project is made impossible by the "chronic" part of chronic illness, but this is also an example of media as capitalism at its most pernicious, when the lived experience of a subject gets sidelined for an imagined experience in order to attract a perceived market of consumers. We are, for example, 3,170-something words into the essay that you are reading right now, and medical science has still not offered any effective means of overcoming any aspect of chronic illness. Yet here we both still are, proving to the world that you don't need to be told how essays will end in order to start reading them.

A third piece was written in response to a request for

essays on medical themes. My pitch was enthusiastically accepted, but the resulting essay deemed "too vague," so I added more science. "Too technical" was the response to the second draft. I was asked to remove details and descriptions as distracting from the story—when in fact we know those often *are* the story. In the end, the piece was not published.

This final response was the most telling. It was an earlier version of this exact essay, a description of my own failure to locate and properly utilize the term *queer crip* to describe my own experiences, as well as a call to revive this moniker, expand the notion of bodily desires from the sexual and particular to the comfortable and general. This time, the editor informed me there was no such thing as a "queer crip"—she was too young to have heard of it, and clearly hadn't bothered to google. On top of which, the term struck her as offensive. If I wanted to be called something, wouldn't it be better to choose something *nice*? she queried. She was certainly willing to run the piece, she explained, but I would have to remove the offensive term that lay at its heart that no one would understand anyway.

Vocabulary, narrative structure, timing, style: at what point shall we acknowledge that it's not the formal elements of prose that make editors and robots alike uncomfortable? Trust me, reader, when I suggest that you might be appalled by the scope and breadth of leftist publications that contribute to the silencing of disability narratives—a condition that makes the technological erasure of people with disabilities that much easier to stomach.

Let's end, however, with a measure of hope: I laughed, and suggest you do too. Do not get me wrong—it is a deeply violent form of censorship to erase crips from your publication, your imagined future, or your vocabulary. But one way that we as a culture can respond to vast gaps in comprehension is through humor. When I say *queer crip*, but you hear *queer crit*, *clear crepe*, *career cryptic*, or *queen creep*, we can both giggle as you explain what you thought you heard. *Queen creep. It's so true!* Any response other than further discussion is damage: silencing what is not understood ensures it cannot be considered, or included, in the future.

Why not instead experience the joy of not understanding something, together?

NORMATIVE BODIES UNUSUAL TASTES

IN A WELL-LIT MEETING ROOM tucked behind Frances Glessner Lee's Nutshell Studies of Unexplained Death stands a wall of glass-encased shelves filled with artifacts of human suffering. They are horrific, yes, although along a somewhat different scale than Lee had aimed to depict with her bloody but informative miniatures displayed in the next room. Here on one shelf is a pair of shoes worn by a man struck by lightning, frayed at point of impact; there a tidy bucket of cremains, near a sharpened blade used in a near beheading. An outrageously malformed dental cast stands out, having been taken from a woman postmortem who died after being stabbed thirty-three times, suffering several knife wounds to the face. The collection offers hard evidence of strange deaths that occurred in the real world, a different aim entirely from the tiny, clue-strewn depictions of same that Lee spent years crafting in diorama form as educational tools for homicide detectives. Proof that death can occur at any time, in the most awful of circumstances, as opposed to a mere warning that it might.

"Does it ever freak you out?" I ask my tour guide, Bruce Goldfarb, gesturing toward the display. He oversees it and the Lee collection at the Office of the Chief Medical Examiner in Baltimore, Maryland.

Goldfarb scoffs. "Of course not," he says, smiling. "Would it freak you out?"

It is a rhetorical question. I had driven six hours to visit the Nutshell Studies, which marks me already as someone who absolutely would not get freaked out about death or the sticky leavings that so often accompany it. Any fan of Lee's, the grandmother-turned-armchair-detective who used her dollhouse-crafting skills to create a series of nineteen mini crime-solving instructionals, thereby helping to establish the field of forensic science, would most assuredly not get freaked out by a charred athletic shoe—even if it still contained a severed foot. Even if that foot were years old, rotted now and stinking.

I'm distracted by the image for a moment on the long drive home, before another intrudes: But what does, I ask myself then. What actually scares me?

♦ ♦ ♦

Close to a century after Lee started crafting her Nutshells, it is still considered subversive for feminine bodies to depict life in any extreme, be they women painters of male figures receiving violent comeuppance or femme movie directors trying to get first horror projects off the ground, and I'm pretty sure this is because they are so rarely offered opportunities to explore the terrain and not because they are freaked out by blood. In 2021, the Center for the Study of Women in Television & Film found that women made up only 17 percent of directors on the 250 top-grossing films of that year, down from 18 percent in 2020 and 19 percent in 2015. The percentage of women working as directors on the top 100 films fell, too, from 16 percent in 2020 to only 12 percent in 2021.[1] We have to go back to 2015 to get a sense of how many of those women directors work in the horror genre: a mere 9 percent that year, the lowest percentage of any film genre.[2] Maybe it's gone up since then? It would surprise me.

Nearly a decade ago I analyzed the content, cast, and crew of seventy-four international horror films for a piece published in *Salon* in 2013.[3] Using data submitted by a handful of enthusiasts given no instructions on what sort of films they might include, I found only 5 percent were directed by women, 7 percent were written by women, and 14 percent were produced by women. On-screen, women were listed as leads in 42 percent of these films, yet appeared to lead plot in 48 percent of them—a seemingly minor difference suggesting that these 6 percent of uncredited leading ladies probably got stiffed. (I mean, of course they got stiffed; these are horror movies. But getting underpaid too? Not cool.)

Of the remaining characters in these seventy-four films, 31 percent were feminine in appearance and 69 percent masculine. (There was only a single identified nonbinary character in any of the films I examined.) Women died with less frequency than men in horror films—44 percent of on-screen deaths are women's—although not enough to make up for the initial gender imbalance of the ensemble: a total of 32 percent of all women characters die, as opposed to only 23 percent of men characters. It's true, in other words, that a woman on-screen in a horror film is more likely to die than a man. (Here are some numbers to back up that other long-standing joke, about race being a major predictor of on-screen death: 70 percent of all characters die in horror films, but only 27 percent of them are white.)

The low bar set for signaling the agency of female characters, the Bechdel Test, is still set too high for almost half the films I analyzed: women characters talk to one another about something besides a man in 52 percent of the films, although many passed on technicalities (women characters discussing masculine demons instead of human men, for example).[4] More than a quarter of the films, 28 percent, contained at least one incident of sexual violence—only a handful of them committed against masculine characters—while 19 percent of the films contained more than one incident of sexual violence. On average, however, there was more than one incident of sexual violence per film, since a few of the films I analyzed used serial rape as a primary plot device. The Bechdel Test did seem a useful predictor for sexual violence in film: movies that passed it tended to have limited rape scenes. However, in a classic perversion of a mainstream trope that still somehow fails to benefit women, the Bechdel Test also serves as an indication of whether or not women are granted agency behind the camera: fewer women worked as writers, directors, editors, or producers on films that pass the Bechdel Test than on films that don't. (Whether this means women are more likely to green-light flat or insulting feminine characters is unclear.) Even more disturbing: on-screen feminine agency is unquestionably punishable by death. Of individual films that contain more women character deaths than men, 82 percent pass the Bechdel Test.

It's fitting, in horror, that the platitudes of daily life be upended—but isn't punishing women who divert their attention from men simply reinstating standard misogynist norms for the sake of entertainment? Movies are often said to offer some escape from reality, with giant spiders, evil scientists, and unexplained phenomena always at the ready to distance us from the news of the day. Yet for women viewers of horror, one wonders what sort of escape is even possible. For despite the infrequency of overgrown-arachnid attacks in real life, sexual violence occurs on-screen in horror films at approximately the same rate as it happens to women in the world every day.

Horror film is a man's world, even if we look beyond the production teams that undergird the genre. The most visible fan base, comprised of internet commenters, film critics, and bloggers, is dude replete almost without exception. Even the cultural imaginary created by the world of horror film, where fears take physical form and may or may not be bested within ninety tension-filled minutes, is constructed by and for men. It's not only the enthusiasts and self-proclaimed experts planting a stake in that fictional world, in other words: there are simply more men granted agency to shape the world of horror, and they populate it with more masculine characters than feminine. And while a man who watches horror films is granted distraction by that world from whatever banal horrors he may experience in his life—the daily grind of a shitty job or difficult relationship is temporarily obscured by, say, an on-screen shark that's been crossbred with a bear and a torpedo—a woman or nonbinary viewer is granted no such respite. Neither is a feminine character: she may behead the hurtling bearshark with as much aplomb as the next dude, but chances are good she's still going to have to fend off some guy pulling his dick out of his pants afterward.

This cursory data analysis suggests that an entire genre of film has cohered around men's fears that somehow manages to ignore everyone else's fears entirely. If we take sexual violence as just one example (although vaginal blood, childbirth, or gatherings of naked women around campfires might also suffice), we can reasonably assume that some of the men, if not most of the men, who write, direct, and produce horror films believe sexual violence to contribute to the appeal of the genre. Now, men aren't experiencing sexual violence as frequently as women characters in these films, nor do men experience rape as frequently as women and nonbinary people do in real life. So the fact that men behind the scenes of horror appear to believe that rape heightens tension is not rooted in their own experience of it. Most women probably agree that sexual violence is, well, pulse quickening, to say the least, and I would never argue for a second that it isn't. But what is clear is that men who make horror films value the impact that scenes of rape and sexual violence can have on their bottom line. Sexual violence, in horror films, is good for business.

Emotional responses to sexual violence may or may not be gendered; I have no idea. We do know that more than one in four undergraduate women in college experience rape or sexual assault, according to Rape, Abuse & Incest National Network (RAINN), compared to only 6.8 percent of undergraduate men.[5] Many students don't report sexual assault, and some don't survive it. Yet quite a few do, which means more women than men have managed to cope with the impact of sexual violence in real life. A far greater percentage than women characters who survive it in horror films, certainly.

What I offer for consideration is this: that perhaps what scares cis men most—as evidenced by the fears we are given to consume as entertainment in the horror genre—may often be things that the rest of us have learned to deal with on a daily basis.

▲ ▲ ▲

I had my hymen slit open with a knife without anesthesia, learned as a child to eradicate deep slivers by slicing along their long edge and lifting the object out—quick, quick! Before the capillaries open and bleeding starts!—and got comfortable early on mouthing off to roomfuls of powerful, rich people two to three times my own physical size. Machine guns are plentiful in places I used to spend a lot of time, so having one pulled on me has never proved alarming, although once I did go too far, got arrested, and spent several hours with no worthwhile language skills in detention in a country with an appalling record on human rights, which was more boring than anything else. I nearly died in Nicaragua, another time in Wisconsin, and several times in Chicago. On two occasions over the course of otherwise pleasant conversations I have come to realize I was dining in the company of a serial rapist; on one, a cannibal.

I don't, in other words, scare easily. Not to say that I don't have a lot of anxiety. But worry and fear are different, intellectually. I chew on my anxieties like gum, let them sit in the back of my mind while I tackle a larger task, try to develop the patterns of my life to decrease or confront them, an internal and analogue form of *Tetris*. Whereas fear—genuine, jolting fear—short-circuits intellectual response entirely. I don't "like" to do anything with it because it is not possible to "like" any aspect of feeling scared. Anxiety is a mammalian response to unpleasant stimuli; fear is reptilian. Honest-to-god fear gnaws at me from the inside and propels me from the outside. I become filled with a dread that supplants all normal physical response at the same time that I am forced away from the situation, whether I flee from a scene of danger or hide in my bed from the door and the phone. It doesn't happen often.

Any half-assed psychologist could provide an explanation for my lack of fear and, believe me, plenty have. There are plausible biochemical causes to cite, too: worn-out adrenals, my medically suppressed immune response, a diet almost exclusively composed of plants. We could even look to technology, always our savior, or to the standard condition of modern American life, wherein many genuine fear-producing events have been limited or controlled. Tiger attacks are said to be on the decline, for example. Serial-killer numbers have also dwindled in recent years, both in frequency of individual attacks and in volume of perpetrators. Yet explanations are only interesting if you, an outsider, hope to categorize an anomaly, aim to reduce the stress caused you by the behavior of the aberrant actor, me. The revelation of root causes provides no means to change the facts of my lived experience, as much as they might ease your mind, and wouldn't interest me if they did. This is important, I think: What would motivate one who lacked fear to seek out a means of accruing it?

Or put another way: Why would I not want to be the kind of person who watches horror movies all the time?

♠ ♠ ♠

We're often told that women don't like horror films because they can't stomach the gross-outs, but it seems more likely to me that they simply crave new experiences. Horror films rely far too frequently on an all-male revue of mad scientists, psycho killers, and evil demons who offer little new to women, many of whom, after all, regularly experience blood gushing out of their vaginas or, less frequently, tiny beings inside their bodies making absurd demands, or rapid bodily changes due to hormone therapy. Women and trans and nonbinary people are often habituated to unwanted sexual advances in the workplace or on the street and subjected to invasive inquiries regarding their sex parts—occasionally delivered under threat of violence—or increasingly accustomed to mysterious diseases with bizarre symptoms that no one can or tries to explain. Many experience the additional daily horror of living in a society so tied to gender norms that every move is restricted, like the use of public restrooms, wearing certain clothing outside of the home, or accessing necessary medical care. Very few horror films come close to portraying the banal terrors faced by people who are not cis men.

So the genre is created and populated by its intended audience. Big whoop. But wouldn't the horror subgenre most readily able to examine the very factors at work—biology, gender identity, skin pigmentation—offer more variety, whether of creators or in the cast? Not really. Body horror boasts a lineup just as heavy with cis dudes as the genre that spawned it. David Cronenberg (*Crash*), Brian Yuzna (*Society*), Frank Henenlotter (*Basket Case*), and Clive Barker (*Hellraiser*) are the cis men most often cited as foundational contributors to the filmmaking form—and for good reason. There's little in *The Fly* (even the 1958 original, before Cronenberg's 1986 remake), *Invasion of the Body Snatchers* (1978), *Deadgirl* (2008), or the Human Centipede series (2009–2015)—each also directed by cis men—that doesn't call to mind those directors and the worlds they've envisioned.

That Yuzna was born in the Philippines and Barker gay, and that rumors swirl regularly about Henenlotter's sexuality, should give us some hope that body horror might allow for a wider degree of diversity and tolerance among its creators than other filmmaking genres, but such hopes wither quickly. Cronenberg and Henenlotter, as well as Marcel Sarmiento and Gadi Harel, codirectors of *Deadgirl*, and Tom Six, the creator of the Human Centipede series, all stand accused of misogyny.

Six, at least, is direct about his negative portrayal of women in *The Human Centipede*. "Politically, it is very incorrect," he explains coolly to *The Guardian* of his infamous film series, in which various unlicensed medical practitioners sew groups of often-female victims together, mouth to anus, in order to see how long they survive when consuming only the waste of the people whose assholes are sealed to their faces.[6] When pressed further on his gender politics in the late *Gawker*'s even later film site, *Defamer*, however, Six is tellingly dismissive of personal accusations of misogyny. "I absolutely love women," he says.[7] One of the characters in the final film—the third, and easily most offensive, of the series—is "an asshole," he concedes. "He's very bad to women. But it's great to write it!"

The warden of the film is a serial rapist, indeed (as well as a murderer and flagrant violator of most civil and human rights), but the charge leveled at Six isn't solely due to this character. In the larger context of this particular film, women have been written out of the script almost entirely, save the warden's sexually abused assistant and a jar full of dried clitorises the warden keeps on his desk and snacks on in times of strife. Yet Six asserts that he is just giving the people what they want. "Horror audiences, they want to be thrilled, they want to be entertained because they are safe, themselves," he explains, in a tone described as "chipper."

It's uninventive, to give people exactly what it is they are thought to want, although it is a popular excuse for boring choices in filmmaking. Harel took a different track with independent film site ScreenAnarchy to attempt to derail accusations of misogyny arising from his portrayal of a group of boys who find a lifeless woman and hide her away for their entertainment. "She was so easy," he says, praising the work of *Deadgirl*'s lead, Jenny Spain.[8] "But she was also chained down."

Harel's joke is both true and funny, but fails as miserably as Six's comments to defend him from placement in the ranks of vile woman haters. In fact, his statement points to the bizarre situation he has created in which a woman is chained to a table and repeatedly raped and mutilated under his direction, for which he praises her.[9] It's even easier to point out that Six's "love of women" is defensive and apparently fair-weather; elsewhere in the same interview, he compares women to mice, and claims he would never hurt either, which beyond the bizarre association makes one wonder what exactly he believes a misogynist does.

Back a bit away from body-horror films in which men and boys commit disgusting evil or stupidity to unseemly ends, however, and the tropes don't change that much. Body-horror films that center feminine characters too often reveal a weird sanctity for the imagined object of desire of your average straight white cis man—the straight white cis woman. Derek Franson's *Comforting Skin* (2011), Jimmy Weber's *Eat* (2014), Eric England's *Contracted* (2013), Norbert Keil's *Replace* (2017), and Chad Archibald's *Bite* (2015) all feature pretty, skinny, white young cis women protagonists who suffer gradual disfigurement. That, for the viewer, is supposed to be the horror: women becoming less pretty. In *Comforting Skin*, the change is minor: lonely Koffie gets a tattoo that comes to life, so she performs a slight self-surgery, off camera, to return to normal. In *Eat*, it's significant: failed actress Novella McClure starts eating bits of her own skin, and soon turns on others before meeting a bad end. While in *Bite*, the change is fantastic: pretty bride-to-be Casey is bitten by an unseen animal on a bachelorette weekend and soon finds herself spawning slimy eggs on every surface of her apartment as she transforms into a hideous amphibious wretch.

This is all fun, don't get me wrong. Watching Casey's fiancé grow increasingly uncomfortable with her prolific new spawning habits is tickling, while the ooze-covered body-morphing orgy Yuzna depicts in *Society* remains a pinnacle of the genre. But it's also all clearly misogynist— not to mention racist and ableist—despite that body horror offers the unique opportunity to explore and subvert physicality like no other form.

♦ ♦ ♦

My diminished fear response doesn't come up often in polite conversation, in truth, although my taste in movies does. In fact, I'm asked all the time why I like horror films, or rather I am frequently accused of liking horror films, and even today in the year of our lord whatever year it is, liking horror films implies something akin to class traitorship. Eyebrows furrow and mouths pucker and questioners visibly balk. "Why?" they ask after I profess my viewing habits, although sometimes in all caps, and with many more question marks: "WHY????" Why subject yourself to an array of fearful situations, imagined and scripted and produced by experts in heightening the most unpleasant emotion?

I confess I have responded by suggesting that it's the genre of film that comes closest to depicting the environment of my childhood home: unpredictable, always creepy, occasionally terrifying, and usually best avoided. It's an easy answer, a capitulation to the many armchair therapists who like to imagine that my pleasure in viewing such films comes from whatever struggle the hero endures before final credits roll, whether she commits a zombie massacre or endures a million rapes before her skin is finally peeled off in long, preserved sheets. Conventional wisdom holds that I identify with the Final Girl, being in fact something of a Final Girl myself, and see in her travails a fictionalized triumph over my own triggers of PTSD.

We're told something similar about the hordes of women devoted to true-crime podcasts, that they're all amateur detectives eager to solve cold cases while the babies nap or the beef roast cooks. I don't buy it. For one, my childhood was odd, but more Netflix-doc odd than zombie-rape odd. And wouldn't my trauma response have shifted or subsided over time if horror movies somehow relieved it? I mean, I watch a lot of horror movies, more than enough to have achieved some sort of effect, but after decades retain pretty much the same triggers I always have, no more or less of them, really—although creepy clown dolls in children's bedrooms never bothered me until I saw *Poltergeist*. (I maintain that my concerns here are primarily aesthetic.) As for the true-crime enthusiasts bored at home with endless domestic chores—doesn't it make more sense that they might be filled with a rage better released through audio mimesis than any other attendant possibility?

Before writing the above paragraph, I'd never listened to a true-crime podcast, mostly because if I wanted to hear people reading Wikipedia entries out loud I would do it myself. So I binged one or two of the most salacious and remained mostly uninterested until an interviewee casually mentioned that she liked horror movies.

It didn't surprise me. Anyone willing to go on a true-crime podcast is more than likely the precise intended audience for all horror movies, but this particular interviewee was filling more of a victim role than a commentating one. As Deborah Elizabeth "Fauna II" Hodel describes it in TNT's *Root of Evil: The True Story of the Hodel Family and the Black Dahlia*—and much of the series is devoted to backing up her claims—she had a childhood most would call truly horrifying. Socially isolated and emotionally manipulated. Regularly raped by her mother, grandfather, and clients of her mother, who took money to send her children out to spend weekends in hotel rooms with strangers. Forced to give birth at fifteen so her mother could increase her child-welfare income. Thankfully, eventually, a teenage runaway. She was even named in part, family lore has it, for her grandfather's most famous victim, Elizabeth Short, because oh! By the way! He was—allegedly—a prolific and infamous serial killer.

What Hodel says on tape is that she watches a lot

of horror movies because she's hoping to find someone whose life is worse than hers. She never has, she admits. But she does not say that she stops watching them. She does not suggest that she has learned now that she will never find anything worse, that after so many years of watching what a largely masculine pool of horror-movie makers thinks is terrifying, she has finally come to realize that her regular daily life as a woman offers the worst imaginable horror.

We tend to ascribe a feminine interest in horror to an innate desire to soothe or heal or resolve, but I'm suspicious of the instinct to explain away a comfort with the macabre with a desire to nurture. My own ease in navigating certain kinds of fear and trauma simply means I can watch a wider array of stories unfold than most people can, with less distress, and I think what might be gendered about this—that is, how I may have interpreted this skill after several decades of life as a woman in American society—is that I sense in myself a responsibility to do so, an urge to see what others choose not to, a willingness to witness causes of suffering. But the desire to see is quite different from the desire to fix.

What I can say about women and horror after several decades of this particular form of witnessing is this: little that can be portrayed on-screen in two hours or less and within a set budget comes close to the banal horrors I watch the women in my life face every day. The single friend in Texas who just discovered she is pregnant, again. The friend who pieced together her husband's pattern of sexual assault too late to save a family member from attack. The friend stuck in a shitty job in a dying industry. The friend whose body has gone haywire and, eight years in, still hasn't found a doctor who can explain why. The friend whose child can't sleep for the active-shooter nightmares. The friend with terminal cancer during a pandemic. The friend laid off from the newsroom with no family and no other marketable skills. The friend whose boss has grown tired of her absence due to long COVID. The friend whose mother claims a new deadly disease whenever she is faced with an unpleasant task. The friend whose partner keeps fucking the interns behind her back. The friend who was fired for whistleblowing. The friend whose new boss was her first rapist. The friend whose transition may soon be forcibly reversed. The friend with unexplained pain whenever she eats. The friend who can't get her autoimmune medication because it is an abortifacient, even though she's been on it too long to get pregnant.

I can't rightfully claim to enjoy horror movies because I have any desire to save myself or others from fictional onslaughts. Like Hodel, I like them because I hope they will someday provide an external, imagined narrative that is worse than what I see or experience in real life. Several decades in, I keep watching them because of how flagrantly they fail at the task.

♦ ♦ ♦

Whether or not women should answer for their likes and dislikes at all is the theme of Julia Ducournau's *Raw* (2016). A coming-of-age protagonist, Justine, first thrown into turmoil over her unusual desires, soon comes to explore them, identify them, and share them with her family. Okay, her specific desires are for consuming the flesh of humans, and I get why that might cause some internal conflict. But what I connect to in this film is Justine's self-acceptance despite the extremes of her physical experience. (Ducournau's next film, *Titane* [2021], takes this internal shift to its next logical step, wherein a woman who really loves cars begins to lose her humanity, although I liked it less because I watch body horror for the bodies.)

A genre established to explore the loss of autonomy, body horror explores bodies of all varieties, often recut or reengineered well beyond the limits of traditional sex, gender, or race—or for that matter nationality, economic class, or even humanity. It is why body horror, when done well, can elicit a physical reaction in the viewer. A film may be visceral because it is vividly depicted, yes, but it also affects our viscera. In Cronenberg's *The Fly*, for example, Jeff Goldblum's character famously becomes twitchier, more harried, and increasingly disgusting as his body gradually transforms into a giant insect. In *Society*, an otherwise dorky 1980s teen-boy-coming-of-age film, the underpinnings of the upper class are revealed: sex parties and mutations and ritual naked acts between close blood relations are contrasted with more banal horrifying bullshit like real-estate deals and country clubs. Often, the "victims" in body-horror films are female, whether the subjects of experiments or the corpses left by previous subjects of experiments. But not always. In fact, we are almost as likely to see a male body mutilated in the horror subgenre as a female body, as much as the bodies of the latter may be singled out for more extreme abuses, discussed in more dismissive terms, or only present under an inequitable pay scale. (In recent months I've noticed something distressing: that body horror that does stray from all-white casting tends to single out Black women's bodies for more extreme forms of abuse. *She Never Died*, for example, Audrey Cummings's semifantastic action/horror title from 2019, features a stunning Olunike Adeliyi as a mysterious stranger able to withstand extreme torture as she saves less-witting victims. But the film lands on a note of torture porn, and not body horror, as viewers are kept from any interior sense of the character's rage and terror, left only to watch her excessive mangling from a remove.)

What remains unwavering about body horror is that, regardless of a subject's race, gender, or class, the subgenre hinges on a notion of normativity. A subject always starts as "normal" and over time becomes "abnormal."[10] Embedded in the assertion of what is normal, we find a set of presumptions about race, of course (and so most of these films are littered with white people), and about gender (so the gender binary is strict and assigned gender roles frustratingly regressive), but also about what roles, behaviors, desires, and appearances are appropriate for everyone.

Twitchiness and excessive hairiness are socially inappropriate, we learn from *The Fly*, and an open fascination with death or dead bodies portends a criminal future, as we see in *Deadgirl*, and thousands of other artifacts from the horror genre going all the way back to Mary Shelley's *Frankenstein*. Biting hangnails is a problem for women, both *Eat* and *Raw* tell us, and as for women who like cars? Sociopaths, *Titane* explains.

These are dismissible lessons, when individually taken, and castigation for ignoring the social contract rarely goes beyond a friendly joke or chiding comment. As a whole, however, body horror's reliance on physical transformation does draw a clear line between the physical human forms we find socially acceptable and those we do not. It is in the assertion of body normativity that body horror most clearly lays out its ableist roots: in depicting the dissolution of normal, that is, the genre does quite a bit to ensure that normal will never change.

This presents a problem of cognition to a person whose body fails flagrantly on a fairly consistent basis. When a knee stops bending for thirty hours without known cause or a wrist becomes inflamed after a day of strain from the untaxing act of reading books, it is less than enjoyable to watch an angelic toddler descend into vampirism, zombism, or the effects of scientific experiment and also be treated cruelly for it. For as much as body-horror films do often visually depict situations that feel familiar to someone who's never quite sure all the limbs are gonna work right all day long, it takes a director like Ducournau to let disability, unusual tastes, and nonnormative desire reestablish what normal might look like when bodies begin to horrify.

Of course, there is opportunity in failure, and it is the persistent failure of normative bodies to maintain their normativity, or even to pretend to want to, that suggests that body-horror films hold the potential to become radical visioning tools. Through body horror, we could explore the possibilities on offer when the abnormal becomes quite common. Think *Night of the Living Dead* recast in the *Cabin in the Woods* universe and managed by Jigsaw, the overseer from the Saw franchise: What if everyone you knew were besieged by a different form of inescapable physical or emotional torture? And what if—continuing the thought experiment for a moment—the daily administration of trauma were totally unremarkable, just something to be dealt with, like laundry and beef roasts?

▲ ▲ ▲

In Jen and Sylvia Soska's *American Mary* (2012), a charmingly gory Canadian film, the daily administration of trauma does become unremarkable. It's even celebrated. The film is quirky, well acted, and unpredictable—a feat in a genre in which pretty much the next thing that will always happen is that someone will die.

There is a rape scene, early in the film, fully contextualized, clearly not employed to contribute to viewer trauma. Compare to the popular but extremely rapey *V/H/S* of the same year, for example, which uses the found-footage conceit to explore six brief tales. Of these, three feature rape or the threat of it as turning points in stories about cis men; a planned sexual assault even acts as a plot device in David Bruckner's installment, "Amateur Night." This is fairly standard in a genre that usually explores the thwarting of cis men's desires, but in *American Mary*, the rape scene is so understated that you may not even notice when it occurs. When Mary later responds to her attacker, with deliberation and focus, it is clear that rape need not act as a given within a larger unfolding narrative of terror. *American Mary* presents sexual assault as event, not consequence.

Following her rape, our protagonist leaves school to focus on independent study once it becomes clear that the price of entry to the aboveground world—in tuition fees as well as in the emotional distress of regular run-ins with her professor/rapist—is too high. This glitch in her plans is made plot by the fact that she's studying medicine: Mary wants to be a surgeon and has no intention of giving up this goal upon leaving school.

Her sexual assault is appropriately traumatic and fully survivable, but the film also offers viewers a female character in horror who retains agency and regains her body autonomy. Indeed, whenever she begins to question her abilities, talent, or value, Mary receives no small amount of positive affirmation for being who she wants to be. She becomes, indeed, a world-class surgeon, highly paid and well-esteemed for her exquisite skill with the scalpel. Unlicensed though she may be, her work in the underground world of body modification is highly sought-after.

Now, Mary is also killing people and mutilating them, or less frequently threatening them feloniously. She's . . . delightfully complicated. Not that there aren't flaws in the film—it's set in Canada, and the characters are Canadian; no explanation for the title unfolds in the narrative— but it's solid. Set design, costuming, and acting are all thoughtful and unindulgent. The genius of *American Mary*, however, is its sharp focus on feminine bodily autonomy in a world that seeks to control and exploit women.

The drama is too calculated to be vengeful and the gore too (ahem) surgical for *American Mary* to be classified as rape revenge. This is simply body horror, in the serial-killer tradition—and centered around a smart, strong lady. A slight precursor to Ducournau, maybe, but worlds away from contemporaries like *Comforting Skin, Eat,* and *Contracted*. Like *Raw*'s Justine, Mary as a physical form never falls out of normative range; she forces other bodies to, and takes great pleasure in it.

Like all media, horror films are formed in the cluttered,

fetid bowels of capitalism, but more than most other forms of entertainment, they remain reliant on the underpaid labor and silence of feminine players (a final nod to *Deadgirl*'s Jenny Spain) to function unhindered. Gender in horror, therefore, always has meaning; gender in body horror—somehow one of the most masculine of the horror subgenres—is often the entire point. In *American Mary*, and in *Raw*, part of what is horrific within the worlds created by the films is that a female character retains autonomy over her own body throughout, eventually taking control over the bodies of others.

It is something, no? A whole subgenre of film intent on depicting the failure of normative bodies, failures most often occasioned by male characters and nearly always fashioned by male directors? (Even in *Bite*, our pretty bride-to-be is presumably impregnated by a male fish before her transformation.) Meanwhile, body transformation is something that women who have been sick or pregnant or had periods or surgery have already experienced and managed to survive, not to mention those who find their daily lives changed in fundamental ways after experiencing sexual violence, or under the systemic labor abuses of capitalist production, or even just existing in a country where the full right to bodily autonomy is granted within a lifetime and then revoked. Body transformation is often unremarkable, too, in transmasculine and nonbinary lives, whether through breast binding, hormone therapy, or surgical operation. And of course in public, where the surveillance and policing of all bodies that fail to conform to a cis male ideal is seeping into more and more sites: bathrooms, libraries, abortion clinics, grade schools, sports teams.

Yet there remain quite a few of us for whom body horror is actually kind of banal. So many, in fact, that if you ask me why I like horror movies, I'll think of Frances Glessner Lee, Deborah Elizabeth "Fauna II" Hodel, Ducournau's Justine, *Deadgirl*'s Jenny Spain, and *American Mary*. And probably just sigh.

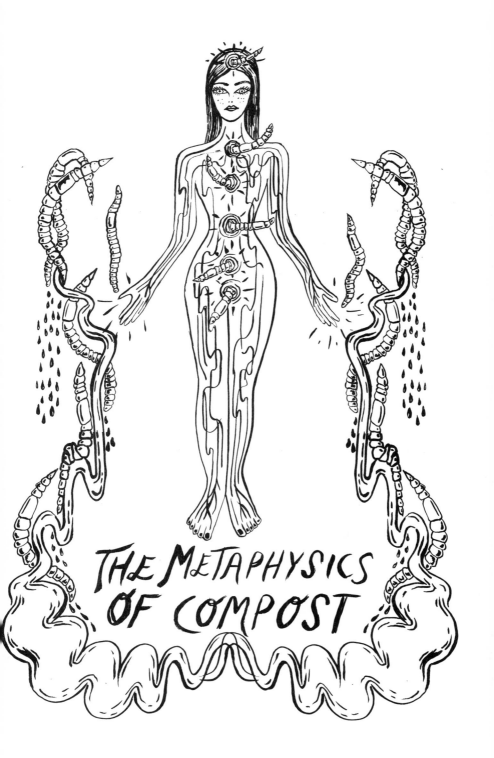

THE METAPHYSICS
OF COMPOST

I DON'T WANT to go into it all over again right now, so let me just start by explaining that I almost died, like, eighteen times a few years back, so I pretty quickly got used to thinking about death in a functional way. Not as something through which I will personally be able to function—that would be ridiculous. Rather, death as an aspect of existence, as a likelihood, even as a future, um, event. One we may never RSVP to on Facebook, but that we will all attend anyway. More interestingly, I grappled at that time with death so frequently, and in such a short period, that I started mulling over ways that it might hold value for me, now, while I am alive. Death as imminent, and not wholly unfriendly. Not to say that I am eager to personally embrace it as a state of being, mind you.

What I am saying is that death—being inevitable, they say—became at some point for me an intellectual banality, a scheduling concern, a daily consideration. Then, shortly after I became slightly bored by the concept, I got . . . intrigued. High school biology classes teach that the cessation of life is the first stage of a whole other process, one that starts with decay and then becomes nourishment, which is life-giving. See where I'm going with this? None of this live-every-day-as-if-it-were-your-last business. More like: *Live every day as if, at the end of it, something new and exciting was going to happen.* I started preparing for death, then, materially as well as emotionally. Not mine precisely, but in general.

In other words, I started a worm bin.

▲ ▲ ▲

My move to a majority Bangladeshi neighborhood in Detroit in May 2016 after more than two decades split between Chicago and various hotel rooms, couches, and flats around the world presented an opportunity to reestablish the foundation of my life without inconveniencing anyone else through divorce, marriage, or birth. I saw the house I was given as a reward for having won the Big Coin Toss as an acknowledgment that my survival had neither been guaranteed nor would it prove to be permanent. So with little fanfare, I packed up my worms, drove five hours east, and dug my new foundation in the unsolid principles of useful decay. It seemed an appropriate metaphor for that particular moment in my life, after several serious health crises, as well as for the city that has come to symbolize urban ruination around the world. Decay not exclusively as *death*, then, but as both the end of life and the future life that ruination fosters. That's the part politicians ignore while warning constituents away from becoming the next Detroit.

I put seeds in the ground before I'd unpacked a single box and found that I had become a gardener. Not merely one who drops a couple beans in some front plots of dirt to see what will happen, although I have the utmost respect for folks who can keep their hobbies in check. I planted seedlings, invested in literature, and joined associations. I bought books—first one, soon a small library. I eschewed my work—writing, I remind myself sometimes—for projects like stump eradication and research into companion planting. Of course, from these efforts naturally emerged the time-consuming lunch experiments, the driving inquiries behind which quickly evolved from "How can I best prepare this vegetable that I recognize and could purchase in the store?" to "This sort of looks like food and did come out of my garden, so I'll just pop it in my mouth and see what happens." *What's the worst-case scenario here, it could kill me?* ran a query through the back of my mind. *Get in line.*

Most significantly, I crafted a compost bin from a couple of concrete slabs in my backyard, and then another slightly larger one next to it. I daily filled one or the other with food scraps and covered those with a thin layer of soil. My chronic illnesses come with an array of food restrictions, so I banned what I couldn't eat from both my kitchen and my compost bin. Conversely, I forged a pact with my coconspirators in this life-cycle project—all microbes, insects, and worms—and eliminated most of what could not be composted from my diet as well. One should never feed anything to friends, single-celled or otherwise, that one wouldn't consume oneself.

I then added a third bin, about two feet wide by ten feet long, for turning yard waste into usable soil. In sum, then, I managed three distinct plots of land, each devoted to meeting requirements for draining all vestiges of life from particular forms of organic matter for, ah, microbial reuse. There was more physical space in my immediate environment devoted to enabling processes of decay than to any of my other obsessions except books.

My composting habits were not even limited to the yard. Indoors, I kept the worm bin, a two-tiered contraption that, in theory, would allow the red wigglers I ordered from the internet to feed on fruit scraps in the top bin, safely nestled in some wet-newspaper bedding, until their home filled with waste and they were forced to move house. Then I would place bedding and food scraps in the bottom bin, and the worms—again, in theory—would make their way through the holes that I had drilled in the bottom of each container to their new abode. The notion was that the two-tiered bin would allow me to make easy use of their leavings.

In reality, however—and this is important to the process, I think—the leavings we are talking about were worm poop, and the worms liked living in it. So when I required some vermicompost, I scooped it out and placed it directly under a seedling. After snuggling that worm waste in next to some food I was hoping would eventually happen, I plucked the worms from it, one by one, with my bare hands, and returned them to their proper locale.

The neighbor girls would screech at this, their parents exclaiming out loud in Bangla at the sight of me digging worms out of some poop that I have just placed next to some vegetables, possibly because they knew I would eventually try to get them to eat those vegetables with their mouths. I did not blame them. It *is* disgusting. There are ways to make the process less disgusting, of course, but I tend to forgo them. They are distractions, I feel, from the process of ensuring that the beings I have enlisted in my agenda of useful decay are well cared for and enjoying their work. I can't say for sure that I knew when my worm friends were happy, of course, but they seemed to like banana peels and being left alone in their bin. They were particularly important to the composting process: their waste is especially nurturing for young plants. I treated the worms with care, therefore, and gave them only the foods they seemed to like, which I gauged by noting how many of them crowded around certain scraps in a wriggling mass, the sight of which cannot be described as anything less than disgusting. Like the snake pit scene in *Indiana Jones and the Temple of Doom*. It played out in my kitchen every day.

It became clear around this time that the world as it existed did not facilitate my survival. What I was doing in Detroit was nudging an entire tiny ecosystem toward a state that would allow my participation, crafting a mini-biome with millions of other beings. My worms were my closest collaborators in this project; an added benefit is that they kept the process visceral. It is one thing to bury food scraps in the backyard, it turns out, and another to keep pooping worms in your pantry. The latter can churn the stomach, which is only appropriate. A whole new ecosystem *should* be felt in the gut.

Both backyard and vermiculture composting captured the imaginations of a growing number of folks alongside a rise in urban farming and the popularity of the sustainable food movement. It is not uncommon to heap a healthy dose of hyperbole in with the food scraps for the backyard bin either: composters tend always to infuse their talk of rot and decay with grandiose notions of life-force sustenance and metaphors for Important World Events.

The *Los Angeles Times* predicted the trend with a short piece of compost boosterism published in 1989, just as the Berlin Wall began to fall:

> Among the several things about which Karl Marx was right is the uncontestable fact that consciousness is determined by one's relationship to the means of production. And what finer method to approach the consciousness of one's garden than to partake in its death and regeneration.[1]

Hyperbolic, maybe, but provable. Among the many rewards of composting listed in the article that follows are the horticultural (of course), the political (which we'll address in a moment), and the metaphysical. I'll personally attest to this last: I know I've never felt more connected to the spiritual cycle of life—the one that exists beyond sight, taste, smell, sound, and touch—than when I am digging around in a delightful pile of rotting gook and poop and death, pondering my own demise with a certain measure of serenity and hopefulness.

▲ ▲ ▲

The metaphysics of compost, according to writer and researcher Kim Q. Hall, is more than just a woo-woo guide to backyard gardening: it may help inscribe justice into a mainstream food movement currently distracted by inherently capitalist notions like sustainability, purity, and consumption. Food often acts as invitation, a means of sharing both physical space and a nourishing—potentially educational, definitely cultural—experience. Considering food within a larger sociocultural context allows us to comprehend it not as a mere site to improve the minutest impact of globalization, but as an easy access point to politics that are rooted in resisting oppression.

Consider that darling of the mainstream food movement, the farm-to-table restaurant. These serve what's often called "pure" food, sourced from local growers in a manner described as "sustainable." Such establishments are often correctly chided as elitist, although farm-to-table eateries pride themselves on crafting healthful meals that provide pleasure.

The charges of elitism aren't tossed out solely over the high cost of locavore dishes: such facilities are often unlikely to respond to individualized food needs, a stance that quickly privileges the able-bodied over those who may have more pressing reasons to seek healthful food options. I've heard more than one server suggest that if I don't "like" ingredient X—one that may trigger pain or dysfunction, but which the chef has determined is a part of how a meal tastes best—I should probably just eat at home. This same suggestion was once offered a friend who has no food restrictions, but is larger framed than I, and who had requested an untiny table that she could more easily access, so even the built environment of an establishment can cater to a particular variety of eater. Many restaurants, too, fail to install ramps for wheelchair access or other devices for mobility assistance, few offer large-print menus for the visually impaired, and I've yet to enter a restaurant that offers American Sign Language as a matter of course. Far from mere oversights (and occasional violations of the Americans with Disabilities Act, or ADA), such tendencies build to a pattern that infuses the mainstream food movement with ableism, centering it on a desire to ward off—instead of acknowledge and respond to existing—disease and disability. (In her essay "Toward a Queer Crip Feminist Politics of Food," Hall reminds us that additive-heavy but cheap fast food is served in ADA-approved facilities and often available for extended hours, which gives us a solid glimpse of why the drive-through may arguably be more "sustainable" for people with disabilities than the average farm-to-table eatery.)

There are grander implications to positioning food as pure, too, even besides the mythos of white supremacy the term calls up. I'll attempt to outline an economic argument based in my own experience. Let's grant a normal, healthy body—one capable of gaining all the nutrients it needs from meals—a weekly food budget of one hundred dollars, and assume that, for the sake of argument, to be standard. Folks with any sort of health concerns, however, are likely to have a diminished ability to process certain nutrients, whether from illness itself or as a side effect of a treatment program. Supplements can be expensive: mine cost approximately $120 per month, or $40 per week. Which leaves me with a starting (imaginary) weekly food budget of only $60. So when food is presented as healthful, but not priced with budgetary diversity in mind, it is targeted mainly toward those who are already free of serious health concerns. The purity of the sustainable food movement, then, is not an attainable state for all clientele: it is granted only to some, before even entering the establishment, and the already pure must guard the state carefully.

Yet everything, we know, must end in decay, and Hall writes of eating, disability, and the myth of sustainability in this context. We are, she reminds us, messy: how we eat and, even more, how we navigate relationships around eating. "Food practices are sites where the meanings of community, identity, relationship, and the meaning of food itself are materialized and negotiated," she writes.[2] The notion of purity, she argues, or even untrammeled longevity, has no place in how we really eat. Even tastes change over time after all.

Food politics that center on justice, Hall contends, would hold the relationships forged by what we eat and how we acquire it as equally important to the nutritional properties of what is ingested. In real terms, the labor practices at that farm-to-table restaurant would come under consideration as another aspect of our health. Does a restaurant that touts sustainability consider providing for its employees as important as nourishing its customers? Is an eatery that fails to respond to the needs of customers with disabilities or food restrictions truly concerned with ecologically necessary biodiversity?

It all comes down to a need to more deeply interrogate the full cycle of food, waste, regeneration, and death, Hall contends, to comprehend "bodies and food as . . . contested sites where boundaries are questioned, negotiated, and open to transformation, not fixed."[3] She urges us to consider food as a complex of relationships. Between my worms, for example, and my neighbors; between me and the microbes that live in my backyard; between local restaurants capable of responding to individualized diets and farmers reliant on sound environmental practices; between the potential interactions that could be formed if high prices and swanky design did not prohibit a diversity of bodies from gathering in any particular locale. (I have taken, of late, to hosting parties in my new home to which no one is allowed to bring other food. Because I wish to ensure others can eat, too, I communicate with each individual in advance of the gathering, requesting dietary concerns and other requests necessary to ensure physical comfort. These are extremely time-consuming activities, true, but they allow for an unusual intimacy to emerge quickly in a roomful of strangers.)

Hall calls for a movement centered, therefore, not on a metaphysics of food, but on a metaphysics of compost. "There are no pure bodies," she writes, summing up her argument for why even food itself should be situated within the ecosystem that supports both its growth and its decay. "No bodies with impermeable borders."[4]

Hall may have been a bit ahead of the game, but the data is now catching up to the theory. In recent years, we have come to understand that human bodies are host to—even made up of—trillions of microbes. We breathe them in, they breed on our faces, we pick them up on the subway or ingest them in the food that we eat. Viruses, too, of course, although science has finally moved beyond germ theory—the presumption that all microbes cause disease—and is beginning to understand that important bodily systems depend heavily on the microbes that inhabit them. The immune system, for example, turns out to rely almost fully on microbes we are not born with, but that we acquire over the course of our lives from other bodies, beings, and plants.

The metaphysics of compost offers a food politics centered on the health and needs of the diversity of beings that contribute to—and turn out to largely constitute—you.

▲ ▲ ▲

Material evidence can be found in Detroit that the metaphysics of compost is not unimplemented theory but daily practice. It is a city filled with friendly people but associated internationally with images of ruin and decay; crumbling buildings are quickly overtaken by vegetation both planned and accidental. My block, largely inhabited by immigrants from Bangladesh, had backyards filled with herbs and vegetables from home countries that most certainly fostered microbial life-forms foreign to my system. (I will note here that these foreign microbes were not only delicious, but kindly intentioned.)

This city is often called to represent failure; in fact, it turns out that narratives about the need to rebuild Detroit have been circulated several times in the city's history, casting it in an impossibly permanent state of decay, fully oppositional to any notion of sustainability. In that, Detroit also points to the flaws of a politics rooted in sustainability, serving as a geographic reminder that all processes do end.

What the residents of Detroit know, and what I experimented with there daily, alongside my neighbors, some worms, and a million friendly microbes, is that decay is not only inevitable but useful, and when it takes place, life can flourish.

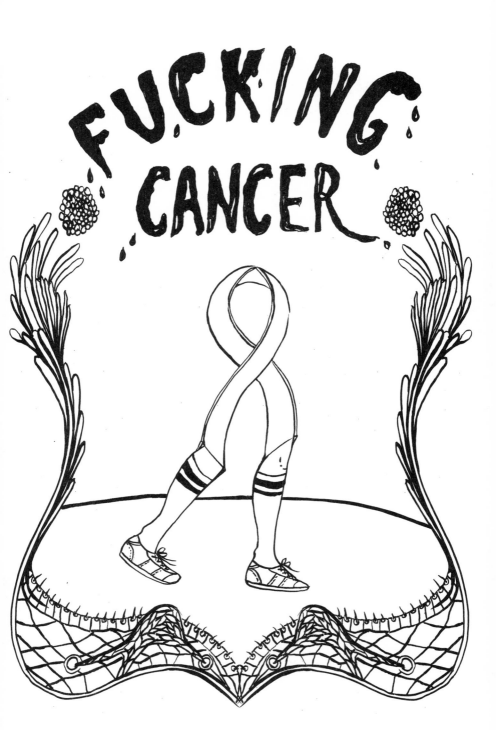

IT'S ELECTION SEASON 2016, and I'm on the elliptical at the gym nearing the end of my workout when I catch the most horrifying ninety seconds I have ever seen on-screen.

About the gym, I should first explain: I go regularly. For a chronically ill person, I'm in spectacular shape. Even on days when I've pushed my body well beyond its capacity to withstand pain, construction workers wax eloquently on the tightness of my ass. The catcalling then becomes more than just a screaming-in-my-face reminder that the patriarchy is doing okay without my emotional support; it reveals itself then to be as maddeningly irrelevant as ever. "*Whooo*—you are doing *great*, honey!" men in bright vests call as I emerge from the facility. *Shows what you know!* I think, viciously, because I am too exhausted to yell.

The flash of satisfaction I get from besting catcallers in my mind is too fleeting to justify an active gym membership. Nor does my beloved sauna explain the devotion—I've encountered too many sincere women doing yoga inside of it and, once, a tidy pile of human excrement. Of course, my body reacts to treatment better and recovers from injury faster when my heart rate hits 140+ bpm three times a week, but even this I consider a bonus. No, I go to the gym because I can fit in some CNN time while on the weirdo cross-country ski machine and, in this way, retain an understanding of what other people think of as politics. Because apparently, not everyone believes that the gendered distribution of medical funding and the resulting limitations that this places on research into the causes of autoimmune disease is the most pressing issue of the day.

On this particular day, someone on the television is saying something about Donald Trump, more than likely the man himself. His video appearance coincides with the hardest part of my workout, so I focus my energy on not vomiting while fake cross-country skiing at a steep incline despite graphic evidence that a reality television star, tax dodger, and self-proclaimed sexual assailant is about to be elected president of the United States. Even *that* is not the horrifying on-screen moment I am about to describe.

When I can focus again a few minutes later, a commercial I've never seen before is fading in from black. It's for Opdivo, "an exciting scientific breakthrough," as a voice-over explains. The sights and sounds of the spot are unmemorable: generic nature; a healthy-looking white man performing a mildly heroic act; an elderly couple gingerly holding hands; soothing, twinkling music. Opdivo, I glean through the reverie, is part of a new class of immune-stimulating drugs that fight cancer.

What's supposed to happen during my five-minute cooldown is that my heart rate should lower from 140+ bpm to something in the mid-90s, but—I test it—it's only rising. Opdivo I know, because I've read about its clinical trials, initiates an autoimmune reaction, so the description of the treatment as *immune-stimulating* jars me. I have between four and seven autoimmune reactions occurring in my body at any given time, and *stimulating* is not how I would describe a single one of them. *Agonizing* comes faster to mind. Also, *debilitating*, *soul crushing*, and *incurable.* There are interesting aspects to these diseases, of course, benefits I could never have imagined in advance. Yet often, there are no words to describe them at all—sometimes because the pain is blinding, and other times because my mind is so muddled with medication I can barely conjure vocabulary.

Drugmakers claim Opdivo coaxes the body's natural immune response into hyperdrive, inciting it to attack cancer cells with as much abandon as my dysfunctional immune system is currently attacking the joints in my right wrist, my salivary glands, the skin on my elbows, and a healthy length of my intestines because someone snuck dairy into the fish I ordered at a restaurant last night despite my clear outline of food restrictions while placing my order. This is stimulating to me in the same way that getting punched in the nose might be stimulating. What the pharmaceutical company only hints at in the small print of this injectable is that once stimulated to attack, the autoimmune response doesn't necessarily stop on command. It may remain stimulated, even if all the cancer cells it was called on to eradicate have been destroyed. (That's why autoimmune disorders are treated like diseases and not like add-ons at the spa.) Even if immune-stimulating drugs do work on the intended target, they may provoke a system of autoimmunity that will go on to attack whatever was lying beneath, near, or beside it: your stomach lining, your blood, or your liver. The autoimmune response doesn't care.

I suddenly feel as if I *have* been punched in the nose. What I am watching on television is an advertisement for some of the exact fucking diseases I am trying, at this moment, to survive.

On an intellectual level, I can see that the logic holds. Harnessing the autoimmune response to fight cancerous growth is theoretically sound—and just the tiniest bit clever. However, medical science has never found a reliable way to reign in the autoimmune response for those suffering its worst effects, nor for that matter for anyone else. Other concerns flare up: Opdivo is approved to treat an advanced-stage lung cancer, renal-cell carcinoma (kidney cancer), and certain melanomas (skin cancers) for which chemotherapy has not proven effective, and thus presents such "immune-boosting" treatments as alternatives to chemotherapy without acknowledging chemotherapy as a first-line treatment for several manifestations of auto-immunity. Here, let me help you out of this frying pan: Opdivo may treat your cancer after chemotherapy has failed, but you may also be stuck with a new chronic illness and even more chemotherapy, in addition to the several serious and lingering side effects of taking the drug in the first place. To me, this all seems a bit counterproductive (but who am I to tell you how to get over your cancer?).

Perhaps most insulting is the expense. A full, twelve-week course of biweekly Opdivo infusion treatments can run as much as two hundred thousand dollars. This is about twenty-five times what I pulled in for the year, a pricey consequence for my particular combination of faulty genes, years of eating preservative-laden food, the occasional course of antibiotics, a high-stress lifestyle, constant international travel, and just regular old Life in the Age of Toxins. If you *really, really* want an autoimmune disorder—and all the cool kids have 'em—why not try a crap Western diet, skipping every third night of sleep, and doing a few shots of Purell? Whole thing'll cost you less than two thousand dollars, for sure. Until you start needing lab tests.

So there I am at the gym, watching CNN condone and install megalomania as New World Order, when a commercial comes on, selling a disease or two that I am desperately trying to keep from doing more damage to my already compromised body. These are ailments I will have for the rest of my life, lit for a commercial audience by soft, white light and accompanied by a lilting tune, and they are going for top dollar. That's not money that will fund research into treating autoimmune disease, of course, but will instead fuel the project of making autoimmunity useful in the treatment of other ailments—proliferating disorders like mine as a result. And all of this is happening before my eyes, at the gym, without a shred of acknowledgment of how difficult, hopeless, and expensive these diseases can be to live with.

When I can breathe again, my first inhale is a gasp. The next exhale is a sob. I begin crying then in horrible jags, angry as shit, my heart rate steadily rising, standing there on that lumbering, awkward machine. I've seen thousands of horror films, but this commercial terrifies me more than all of them combined.

♦ ♦ ♦

The 2014 film *Creep* opens with a bright-eyed, if slightly skittish, videographer arriving at a mysterious freelance assignment he picked up online. Aaron (Patrick Brice) has been offered one thousand dollars in exchange for a day's footage and "discretion." Josef (Mark Duplass), who posted the ad, clears up the mystery straightaway: "I am a cancer

ANNE ELIZABETH MOORE

survivor," he says, describing a prior successful treatment. "Unfortunately two months ago . . . brain tumor, size of a baseball." Josef claims the reappearance of his cancer means he has only two or three months to live. The video Aaron will shoot, a daylong document of Josef's life, is intended for Josef's unborn son.

Aided by the found-footage conceit of the film (we are watching Aaron's video), the videographer's anxiety, and Duplass's overearnestness, the viewer is led on an eye-widening excursion of tiny scares over the course of the two men's weeks-long relationship that never seems to build to larger horror. That is, until just over halfway into the film, when it becomes clear that Josef probably isn't sick in the precise way he claims to be.

Horror films reflect society's deepest fears in absentia; that is, the presumptions that underly the safe version of the world that is destroyed in most horror films are often more telling than the scare tactics utilized by whatever monster inflicts the destruction. Good horror movies exploit presumed bastions of comfort, universally held beliefs that, throughout the course of a film, we may come to understand are built on faulty or wholly false presumptions. *Creep* is a horror film—and quite a good one—based on the premise that cancer survivors are all of a type: they love and value life, are always truthful, and intend no harm. The inverse is also held to be true: that one does not lie about having the disease, that doing so is a violation of the highest moral order. *Creep* shows us someone inherently good and kind—but gullible—who deserves and receives punishment precisely because he believes the best of someone who claims to be dying of cancer.

The plotline calls to mind Susan Sontag's 1978 essay

286

"Illness as Metaphor," which catalogs an affliction she was suffering, albeit through a critical historical overview of disease narratives and not at all as a memoir. The narratives she explores, she argues, create unhelpful metaphors, story lines patients must rail against in lieu of their actual illness-causing agents. Sontag casts disease metaphors as dangerous, energy-wasting distractions from medical treatment that do far more harm than good.

Although publication of her original essay caused medical practitioners, psychotherapists, and naturopaths the world over to throw several hissy fits throughout the ensuing decades—most acknowledging that the hopefulness at the center of many disease metaphors does seem to aid healing—Sontag's point still holds. Her ailment/muse, companion/foe was a disease around which many narratives have been constructed. In fact, there have been so many that there has come to be a standard cancer narrative: beloved figure grows mysteriously ill and fights vainly yet perishes, and the rest of us gain lessons about the value of life from the experience. There have even come to be standard narratives for particular forms of cancer—an unjust and cruel man is afflicted with an aggressive and untreatable cancer; an innocent child remains hopeful in chemo despite overwhelming odds. Individuals are said to be either standard or nonstandard cancer patients, just as particular diseases are thought to behave in particular ways among particular populations. An evil CEO who is unkind to employees and unfair in his business dealings with painful stomach cancer may elicit headshakes if little in the way of sympathy. A healthy, vibrant athlete facing radiation therapy is discussed in almost mystical terms, as if cancer does not regularly afflict the physically fit, and the patient being treated for lung cancer who never smoked a day in her life is thought to have been done a grave disservice. The metaphors all craft a sense of awareness without actual knowledge: Cancer, we feel, is known. Cancer sufferers are known. Cancer survivors are known. The manner in which we respond to cancer survivors is known. The negative medical impact of all this knowing—a vague sort of concern, absent of curiosity—was Sontag's subject.

Although the medical field has advanced significantly since the original publication of "Illness as Metaphor" in the *New York Review of Books*, Sontag's basic assertion still holds true. That we automatically react to the specter of cancer with patience, kindness, and respect is so deeply baked into our culture that responding with questions or criticism would be unthinkable. It is neither my intention, nor was it Sontag's, to challenge an inherently humane response. But we should note that cancer comes to operate, culturally, as a safe harbor: the metaphors still in use to describe the course of the disease—and, in truth, to describe many similar-acting diseases—are reliable, somber, and predictable, however much the diseases themselves continue to defy true knowledge. This becomes tautological: when we treat dangerous elements of any kind as if we already comprehend them, we actively deny ourselves the opportunity to acquire new information about them.

The metaphors of disease can establish a culturally reinforced ignorance of its true dangers and mechanisms, Sontag argued rightly. If you don't believe her, try telling the next guy who says he has a brain tumor the size of a baseball to "Prove it." *Creep*'s Aaron didn't, and I'm not even going to tell you how horribly that turned out for him.

▲ ▲ ▲

When intellectual femmes become ill, they turn, invariably, to Sontag. This does not mean, apparently, that they all *read* her. An overview of literature referencing her work on illness reveals the most quoted passage to be the sly joke from its opening lines: "Everyone who is born holds dual citizenship, in the kingdom of the well and in the kingdom of the sick. Although we all prefer to use only the good passport, sooner or later each of us is obliged, at least for a spell, to identify ourselves as citizens of that other place."[1]

It's the one solid, original metaphor we can pull from Sontag's groundbreaking work—by authorial design. She references the easy glitz of the image herself in the introduction to the book version of her 1988 *New York Review of Books* essay "AIDS and Its Metaphors," released as *Illness as Metaphor and AIDS and Its Metaphors* in 2001. "I prefaced the polemic against metaphors of illness I wrote ten years ago with a brief, hectic flourish of metaphor, in mock exorcism of the seductiveness of metaphorical thinking,"[2] she writes, before acknowledging that metaphors are central to intellectual activity.

Not all metaphors, she responds to detractors from the wellness field. But her point, she goes on to explain, was to review the literature that first set these metaphors in print. She wanted to avoid another first person autobiographical tale of yet another triumphant cancer survivor. She wanted to outline a concept, she writes, not tell a story. It was a project undertaken not to hide her personal narrative in a literary review, but to offer a cultural corrective. "The metaphoric trappings that deform the experience of having cancer," she writes, ". . . inhibit people from seeking treatment early enough, or from making a greater effort to get competent treatment. The metaphors and myths, I was convinced, kill."[3]

Time has since proven a good number of her assertions correct, and many cancer treatments popular in the late 1970s were abandoned or improved in response to the concerns raised in her book. Breast-cancer treatments, for example, became more localized and less invasive as researchers and patients alike began demanding more accurate, individualized responses to the disease. As medicine progressed, it became clear that there was not, in fact, a cancerous personality, a theory popular when Sontag was diagnosed; the evil were not stricken with the disease because they had erred (and would therefore succumb to it), and the good were not immune (and would therefore be cured if they mistakenly fell ill). The metaphors and myths surrounding cancer, without a doubt, caused a great many deaths that could easily have been prevented, as scientific breakthroughs fostered a more accurate understanding of the causes and treatments of various forms of cancer. It is consistent with Sontag's authorial intention. The focus of the patient, the healthcare team, and those who seek to describe the diseases in question, she argues, should stay focused on evidential fact and medical research. Period.

Without going full-bore counterintuitive on you, I'd like to suggest that, today, those with a more proliferative disease than even cancer may be suffering from the opposite dilemma. With autoimmunity, it is the *lack* of metaphors and mythology surrounding these diseases that kills. Some may even be dying in service to the cancer research that Sontag so rightly championed.

♦ ♦ ♦

A description of the popular milieu surrounding autoimmunity is easy enough: a brief overview of contemporary literature is extremely brief, indeed. Minus self-help books and blogs—of which, in truth, there have been a great many—we're left with surprisingly few references, whether literary, journalistic, or popular, for a set of disorders also considered epidemic.

Even Laurie Edwards's *In the Kingdom of the Sick*, a 2013 cultural history of chronic ailments named for Sontag's joke about illness metaphors, strangely offers little to no deep thinking on the subject; neither do the handful of unnamed diseases littered across sci-fi narratives that seem, often, to imply autoimmunity. Donna Jackson Nakazawa's 2008 nonfiction book, *The Autoimmune Epidemic*, pays more engaged attention to the topic (occasionally too much—I cried heartily out of naked fear that each horrendous disease described would be the next to appear on my hospital chart) and is an excellent read of case studies and medical theory surrounding autoimmune conditions. For a time, it fostered in the press a mild interest in the rise of autoimmunity. This died out quickly— faster even than folks perish of Bellini's lymphocemia in season one of Fox's sci-fi series *Fringe* (2008–2013). The fictional autoimmune disease is inflamed by anger, and causes people's heads to explode.

If you want metaphors for autoimmunity, you will find them most frequently on television, particularly on the Fox series *House* (2004–2012), where the diagnoses are often first assumed and then immediately rejected by the eponymous Dr. House. Lupus, notoriously difficult to diagnose, even became something of a running gag on the program. "It's never lupus," the pill-popping sociopathic physician mutters more than once to his hapless medical team as they brainstorm various causes for ailments. The phrase became the program's unofficial tagline, then a meme, then a joke that spread throughout pop culture. As Sontag noted, such jokes have real-world effects. This one became an ever-ready cultural dismissive for a disease that predominantly affects low-income women and people of color—groups that often have trouble accessing health-care services and even more trouble being taken seriously within the medical system. Did the proliferation of the statement "it's never lupus" spur these high-risk populations toward early or competent treatment? Not likely.

"What's Graves' disease?" Kate Micucci asks a weed dealer in the first (and only) season of IFC's 2014 women-led comedy, *Garfunkel and Oates*.

"Oh, that's what you get if you're a grave robber and you go in and you take the body for some sort of nefarious, scientific purpose, and then you find out that you have some sort of fungal infection on your finger," the weed dealer replies. Besides the wordplay, the joke hinges on the fact that Graves' causes anxiety-producing hyperthyroidism, suppressible by marijuana smoking. I guess it's funny?

Autoimmune diseases are played for only slightly fewer laughs in *The X-Files*, another Fox program that originally ran from 1993 to 2002. In an episode toward the end of the second season, a string of characters are diagnosed with Creutzfeldt-Jakob disease, a degenerative neurological disorder thought to be related to autoimmunity. In this case, the disease resulted from the consumption of chickens from a commercial processing plant where feed consisted of human sufferers of the disease who were murdered to cover up the . . . well, it gets a little confusing. The episode ends with a bizarre, colonialist depiction of tribal cannibalism in New Guinea, scary masks and all, lending autoimmunity an exoticized provenance that has no basis in reality but a frisson of terrifying racism.

In the sixth season of Showtime's *Nurse Jackie* (2009–2015), Edie Falco's titular character treats a patient with only a tote bag full of medications for ID. The woman turns out to have a host of autoimmune diseases, and Jackie—habitually drug-addled herself—turns solemn. The patient's sole problem turns out to be medical incompetence: she's been prescribed multiple prescriptions for multiple diagnoses with no centralized oversight. "Not one of her doctors came down," an emergency-room nurse explains to Jackie. "I'm on hold with the rheumatologist right now."

The nursing staff tricks the physicians into a group consultation by telling each respectively that their mothers have just been admitted to the hospital—unethical, perhaps, but based on my experience, a believable depiction of what it might take to get various specialists together to address a single patient's panoply of autoimmune conditions. The episode ends before any incisive medical advice is handed out, but the characterization of autoimmunity as deadly serious but complex beyond the abilities of modern medicine is clear.

BBC's *Orphan Black* (2013–2017) provides one of the more compelling depictions of autoimmune disease in popular culture. An untold number of clones—some kind of corporate-government invention—are programmed with an endometriosis-like disorder to prevent pregnancy that, unfortunately, appears to spread and turn malevolent in the body of each clone. The search for the cure is a journey of self-discovery for each of the identical victims, of course, as well as a cloak-and-dagger intrigue replete with military, scientific, and private-business interests all competing to conceal, nab, or supply knowledge about the clones' diseases, genesis, and creators. That disease was programmed into the clones' design seems a fitting acknowledgment of real-world conspiracy theories about autoimmunity; few medical, scientific, or holistic explanations make as much sense. (Some suggest, in fact, that autoimmune-adjacent Lyme disease *is* a government invention that leaked from a military water source, while the infamously contentious Agent Orange is, in fact, autoimmune in nature.) But that the diseases on *Orphan Black* are mysterious, suddenly triggered, serve the functional purpose of controlling a secret government invention, and appear throughout much of the series to be incurable does little to dispel the myth of autoimmune disease as unfathomable, uncontrollable, and impossible.

In sum, popular representations of autoimmunity are almost wholly consigned to sci-fi and comedy television—even those that have been acknowledged by the medical establishment now for decades. Or longer! These are diseases of the future, the metaphors run, both incomprehensible and ridiculous. And that's where the metaphors stop.

▲ ▲ ▲

The impossibility of knowing autoimmunity to the same degree that we know cancer, it turns out, is a metaphor with a history. German physician and scientist Paul Ehrlich set the theory in motion in the early 1900s with his research into the immune system. You may be surprised to hear that, after much research and a great many cigars, the great scientist—who did, after all, develop the first effective treatment for syphilis—decreed that autoimmune disease could not possibly exist. Then he won the Nobel Prize.

Ehrlich's 1898 experiments led him to his theory of horror autotoxicus, which Arthur M. Silverstein describes in the journal *Nature Immunology* as "the unwillingness of the organism to endanger itself by the formation of toxic autoantibodies."[4]

Ehrlich's precise judgment of the concept of autoimmunity, noted by Silverstein, was that it was "dysteleologic in the highest degree"—fully purposeless, without function. (As someone who experiences daily the ridiculousness of autoimmunity, I don't disagree, even if the makers of Opdivo probably would.) When called on in later years to respond to emerging evidence that, however purposeless, autoimmunity did in fact exist, Ehrlich dug in his heels. Horror autotoxicus, the scientist explained, did not prevent antibodies from forming against the self. That would be impossible! It merely kept autoantibodies "from exerting any destructive action," as Silverstein put it, underscoring Ehrlich's own vague explanation, "by certain contrivances." Thus, Ehrlich dispelled the possibility of autoimmunity for good. At least in his mind.

"Ehrlich's absolute dictum that autoimmune disease cannot occur would resound throughout the decades and prevent full acceptance of a growing reality," Silverstein contends. As recently as 1954, despite scientific reports pointing to the emergence of at least six distinct autoimmune disorders, horror autotoxicus was still considered a law, with holdings as absolute as the law of thermodynamics or those set out by Newton to describe motion. "The ruling immunochemical paradigm" is how Silverstein more democratically refers to Ehrlich's now disproven theory of horror autotoxicus, noting that the possibility of autoimmune disease was still an open question in the 1960s and barely being addressed as a medical reality in the 1970s.

How could an inaccurate (and wholly unprovable) theory hold such sway for so long? In short, the immune system was thought to contain within it a range of emotional responses—aggression, clearly, as well as acceptance—and one of them was horror. The sheer terror the body would naturally feel at the possibility of self-attack was presented as the medical reason autoimmunity was impossible. The logic of this must have seemed, at the time, unassailable. There is no biological reason for a human body to self-destruct: it is, truly, dysteleologic in the highest degree. I can personally barely imagine it, and my inability to imagine it *should* by all *rights* be mirrored in my body's inability to perform it. Except that my right wrist and left foot are swollen and achy today—bodily evidence that, much as I would love to believe him, Ehrlich was wrong.

The idea of the immune system turning on itself *is* terrifying. It is one thing if your guards fall asleep on the job, but once the knights start invading your castle, what's a king to do? Call a meeting to remind them of their duties? Throw the knights an appreciation party? The king would be lanced immediately. It is the combination of the terror of the idea, I think, and the easy accessibility of an existing and at one point quite popular medical theory to justify it, that mounting evidence of the existence of the auto-immune response throughout the twentieth century was ignored or considered aberrant to the "truth" of horror autotoxicus.

Autoimmunity went unacknowledged for generations, not because it was too horrible to consider, but because it was assumed to be so thoroughly terrifying that *the body couldn't possibly allow it*. We believed our biggest fears were impossible, and there's something quite charming in that. As much as I'm aware that this is why no drugs have been developed that can keep my hand from hurting as I type, something deeply trusting lies at the base of this falsehood. It's only too bad how much damage the false-hood continues to cause.

$$\spadesuit \ \spadesuit \ \spadesuit$$

The inexplicable and rampant growth of cells might be considered fascinating, if you have never seen the effects of it in yourself or others. Certainly, the cultural response is fascinating. We talk about beating cancer, run a Race for the Cure, buy pink to fund cancer research. We say, "Fuck cancer!" and we mean it. The fight against cancer is a narrative that we are familiar with and that we invest in, both financially and emotionally. Color-coded ribbons and sympathetic head-shaving rituals are among the ways we indicate to one another: here is a battle that must be sustained, and here is the side upon which I have chosen to fight. The metaphors may not always be apt, or terribly effective, but they act as scaffolding for further exchange. Even Sontag eventually conceded that such metaphors acted as "the spawning ground of most kinds of understanding."[5]

Unlike the community that rallies around you if you are diagnosed with cancer, some prescription pills for the treatment of cancer are quite toxic; if you touch them, you must wash your hands immediately afterward. Because ingesting a drug without touching it can look ridiculous, I sometimes explain to people when I toss back a few pills directly from the bottle, "These are chemo meds." I say this to avoid looking like a crotchety pill-popping sitcom character knockoff—like Dr. House—but my statement has no calming effect. Immediately, whoever I am with will look concerned, or sad, or alarmed. Until I add, "Oh, I don't have cancer," and then they look relieved. Then everything proceeds as if nothing unusual had occurred. As if there was nothing wrong, as if there was nothing else to know.

Like cancer, autoimmune disorders are also fascinating; they are less about the quantity of cells than their behavior. They do not habitually create inexplicable growths: they incite cells to attack any available cells they can find. This is what makes autoimmunity the perfect response to cancer: an autoimmune system will attack until there is nothing left, neither attackee nor attacker. Autoimmunity offers unrelenting but often invisible violence: the sick don't always appear ill, diseases may lie dormant for years before emerging through vague and common symptoms, and tests are administered only once patients complain—or rather, once these complaints are taken seriously, which often takes years of complaints.

Little is known, thanks in large part to Paul Ehrlich, about why these diseases start, how they function, or what triggers them. What is known is that they cause disability, dysfunction, and death, by which I do not mean that they are all fatal—in fact, the number one cause of death of those who've received an autoimmune-disease diagnosis is suicide.

The most significant source of frustration for the afflicted is how few effective treatments have been developed to respond to autoimmune conditions, which is why most of the drugs prescribed have other primary uses. One I took for a while prevents malaria; another, that I did not take, is just gold, injected into the muscles. (I don't know how this came to be a treatment for autoimmunity, but because I like ridiculous things and was willing to try anything, I requested it. My doctor refused to administer it to me, saying it sounded "stupid, like it came out of a comic book.") No one knows why most of the front-line autoimmune drugs work, in fact, because no one fully understands why the immune system goes haywire in the first place. The chemo meds, for example, are simply thought to throw the body into such extreme distress that it stops attacking itself. If you need these drugs, you quickly get the sense that you should feel lucky anyone bothered to find any treatments that help at all.

The National Institutes of Health (NIH) funded auto-immune disease research at slightly under $1.1 billion in 2020—the highest-funded year ever and an increase over 2017's $934 million. Funding has dropped by about $32 million since then, although diagnoses have not: these rise between 2.5 percent and 6 percent per year, depending on the condition. Today, an estimated 23.5 million Americans suffer autoimmune conditions, according to the National Institutes of Health, although the Autoimmune Association, in its previous guise as the Autoimmune Related Diseases Association, suggested this number was a vast underestimation considering the length of time many experience symptoms prior to diagnosis.[6] At 50 million diagnoses, an increase of 2.5 percent would mean 1,250,000 new cases; an increase of 6 percent would indicate 3 million more cases.

Far more funding, of course, goes to the study of effective cancer treatments. In 2020, the NIH dedicated over $7 billion to cancer research, representing a healthy increase over 2017's $5.9 billion. This number continues to rise. In fact, an estimated half billion dollars has been added to the annual budget in the last couple of years. Yet new cancer diagnoses didn't increase much during that time—there were 1.8 million new cases in 2020, compared to 1.7 million new cases in 2017, according to the American Cancer Society. An increase of approximately .1 percent.

Note, please, that funding for autoimmune disease isn't even substantial enough to effectively track the number of new diagnoses on an annual basis. Yet even the most conservative estimates suggest that around one in seven Americans will develop autoimmunity over the course of their lives. Only one in twenty, according to the National Center for Health Statistics, will receive a new diagnosis of cancer, research for which was funded in 2020 at around seven times the budget granted autoimmune-disease research.

In this way, understudied diseases that might afflict as many as fifty million Americans *are* researched, although primarily for their potential to be used by the makers of drugs like Opdivo to treat the cancers of some eighteen million Americans.[7] Sontag's initial concerns clearly still hold true. The metaphors we use to describe illness limit our imaginations—and they hold back or stop still the political force and funding pools required to develop effective responses to rapidly spreading illnesses. But the mythology of cancer Sontag explored was rich and elaborate, particularly when compared to autoimmune disease, about which little to nothing is known.

Cancer is known, while autoimmune disease remains seemingly unknowable. Yet the unknowable has use, it seems, when put to service of the known.

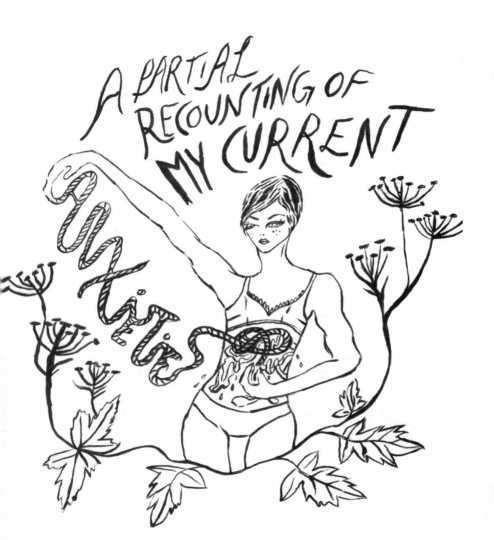

THE CORONAVIRUS. People who aren't worried about the coronavirus. People who are too worried about the coronavirus. The possibility that I am not worried enough about the coronavirus. Case counts. The reliability of case counts. The vaccines. People who aren't vaccinated. The reasons people aren't vaccinated. Getting vaccinated. The mRNA vaccines. My thyroid gland, thrown into disarray by the mRNA vaccine and apparently increasing my blood pressure to dangerous levels. Convincing a pharmacist in a rural red county to give me a booster that is not an mRNA vaccine. Convincing a pharmacist in a rural red county to give me a booster at all. Convincing a pharmacist in a rural red county that the coronavirus is real. Convincing a pharmacist in a rural red county to give me a booster as an immunocompromised person. Explaining to a pharmacist in a rural red county what being immunocompromised means. Convincing my doctor that the mRNA vaccine caused my thyroid disruption, the first I've experienced in over a decade, occasioned exclusively and to the day by my second mRNA vaccine booster. A new coronavirus strain. The effectiveness of masks. Buying more masks. Masking at outdoor gatherings. Transmission at outdoor gatherings. Outdoor gatherings. Being around other people. Not being around other people. The large and embarrassing zit that emerged on my cheek a few days back despite the fact that I am an adult, wash frequently, and do not consume sugar. My autoimmune diseases. The medications for my autoimmune diseases. The vitamins and supplements I take to counteract the medications for my autoimmune diseases. The likelihood of accruing more autoimmune diseases. The likelihood of accruing other diseases because of my autoimmune diseases. Being immunocompromised during a pandemic. Buying clothes during a pandemic. Going outside during a pandemic. Remaining inside during a pandemic. My left forefinger, currently swollen. My blood pressure, still high. My concentration, largely shot. Oh man, a buncha stuff. So much stuff!

What comes flooding in when I have a moment to breathe. The dead tree outside my window, and the path it will take when it falls. Mowing the lawn. Trimming the lawn. The survival of the monarch butterflies. What will happen to my cat if I don't take her to the vet soon. What will happen to my cat if she keeps eating leaves from my fig tree. What will happen to my cat if I have a heart attack. Writing a will. Finding someone to sign my will as a witness who won't freak out about my impending death. Refinishing my furniture in a pleasing enough manner that the beneficiary named in my will won't just throw it away. The calcium supplements I have been taking, triple the recommended dosage, which turns out to cause high blood pressure. New lab results. More lab tests. Where to drop my sharps container. Paying for lab tests. My dwindling grant funding. Inflation. Winter heating bills. Utilities costs. Author-website maintenance costs. The cost of a new computer. Word processing software subscriptions. Book prices. Food prices. Cat food prices. Finding time to run. How running will affect my achy right knee. How running will affect my left leg. Not finding time to run.

Where I can go to swim. Where I can go to swim during a spike in case counts. Focusing on my personal physical health during a global health crisis. Going out to eat with my food restrictions. Going out to eat during a period in American history where setting boundaries around personal health is unwelcome. Cooking for myself, again. Another new coronavirus strain. A new vaccine. Getting the new vaccine. This sore throat. This persistent cough. This fatigue. This diminished capacity to smell. This negative coronavirus-test result. Coughing in public after a negative coronavirus-test result. Coughing in public for any reason. People casually mentioning that they just tested positive for the coronavirus but feel fine. People who would never test for the coronavirus but clearly do not feel fine. This essay. Other essays. Writing. Not writing. Publishing. Not publishing. The publishing industry. The state of this nation's democracy, such as it is. The avowed white supremacist who lives down the road. The Civil War reenactor up the block. The guy at the edge of the village with the flag outside his house that reads, "TRUMP 2024 FUCK YOUR FEELINGS." The guy on the internet who tells me my feelings don't matter. The guy on the internet who tells me I am stupid. The guy on the internet who responds to every post by telling me how hot I am. The guy on the internet who tells me he knows where I live. That my house sits on a hill that is visibly eroding. The oxycodone manufacturing plant in my village. The environmental repercussions of the oxycodone manufacturing plant in my village. The social repercussions of the oxycodone manufacturing plant in my village. The sheer volume of oxycodone that passes through this village. The sheer volume of guns within a five-mile vicinity of my home.

How the vast majority of gun owners in this village fundamentally disagree with me on most basic matters. Not owning a gun. Owning a gun. A civil war. The current Democratic president. Any potential future Republican president. My blood pressure, now both too high and too low. Weaning myself off blood pressure medication. Getting enough calcium in my food without consuming dangerous supplements or dairy. The vitamin D supplements I have been taking too frequently, another cause of high blood pressure. How to get more vitamin D without supplements. Finding time to google every single thing I need to know more about just to survive the week. Remembering to google everything I need to know about to survive the week. Google knowing too much about me. Amazon. Amazon's influence over publishing. Amazon's move into housing. Amazon's move into healthcare. That the calcium supplements I was taking at three times the dose I ordered and which substantially contributed to my high blood pressure were due to an Amazon shipping error. My Amazon rankings. Sales numbers of my current book. Sales numbers of this book. Sales numbers of my next book. Finishing my next book. Finishing this book. Writing books. Reading books. The surprise bill I just got for something that should be entirely covered by my insurance. Calling the insurance company, who tells me to call the billing department. Calling the billing department, who demands I call my RN. My RN, who was fired for refusing to get vaccinated against the coronavirus and then rehired after a couple of months out of desperation and who never got vaccinated. Calling back the billing department, who failed to file my paperwork with the insurance company because they were "too busy" and who asks me to file it myself. That my very complicated disease-maintenance program relies entirely on a medical facility who will charge me three hundred dollars for a fully covered five-minute doctor visit because they're "too busy" to send the same paperwork to someone else. *Dobbs v. Jackson*. The women I know who will be affected by *Dobbs v. Jackson*. The nonbinary and trans people I know who will be affected by *Dobbs v. Jackson*. All the people I will never meet because of how severely their lives will be affected by *Dobbs v. Jackson*. Whether my political organizing in response to *Dobbs v. Jackson* will impact my own political career. Whether or not I can have a political career in a world where people with uteruses have no bodily autonomy. Whether or not I want a political career in a world where people with uteruses have no bodily autonomy. Whether or not I want to live in a world where some people have no bodily autonomy. The kind of people who want to live in a world where some people have no bodily autonomy. Republicans. Democrats. Being told to vote in response to bad policy. Being told to vote by a political party that has more money than god. Being told to vote by the people I voted for. Being told to vote in a world where voting rights are being stripped away from increasing numbers of people. That two out of four times I have tried to vote in this village I have been told I could not. This sudden, inexplicable grief that has no identifiable origin and no end, but some days recedes while I am in the shower and stays in the background for a while, perhaps days, but at other times emerges while I am washing dishes or doing yoga or placing a forkful of salad in my mouth and causes intense chest pain and sudden tears and colors everything gray and that no amount of crying or meditating or talking to friends or sitting in the woods can alleviate in any way. Why my sunflowers have not yet opened. What is going on with my beans. The organic content of the soil in my garden. Why my herb bed isn't filling out. Why my plum trees keep dying. What to do with all this compost. Where to get more raised beds. Wild parsnip. Buying a chain saw. Using a chain saw. Accidentally killing someone with a chain saw. And then wanting to do it again. Purposely murdering someone with a chain saw. Running for elected office. Running for elected office and then having nude pics unearthed on the internet. The kinds of people who run for office. The kinds of people who will never, ever run for office. The weird tendency my left leg has after I've been walking for a mile or so to sort of peter out, to stop performing at peak function, to bend less easily and not lift as high with each step, and how this appears to be a neurological, not a physical, symptom of my medications. Any neurological disease or symptom. Long COVID. Catching the coronavirus as an immunocompromised person and passing along a mutated strain. Accidentally killing someone—oh wait, that's already listed. Mpox. Pretty much all straight white cis men. Straight white cis men who want to play devil's advocate. Straight white cis men who just want to ask me one question about feminists. Straight white cis men who assure me they're not racist. Straight white cis men who speak only to other straight white cis men. Introducing straight white cis men to one another in a professional capacity given the likelihood that they will develop some kind of lucrative project together, leaving me out entirely, often forgetting they ever knew me, that I introduced them, that I used to be their friend. Introducing straight white cis men to music I like. When straight white cis men express interest in my work because they are working on a similar subject. People who too aggressively want to befriend me. Obviously also people who have no interest in me. Engaging with elders in the community during a pandemic. Engaging with elders in the community in a collegial manner and immediately being treated as a sycophant. Becoming an elder in the community. Aging. Trying to behave as normal. Behaving as normal. Trying to remember what normal was. What normal was. The inexplicable knot in my stomach when I wake up every day that takes several hours to dissipate but seems really out of place because actually right now everything is fine, you know, relatively speaking. My dreams, which are often just more of the same. Sleeping, therefore. What will happen next. What will not happen next. How we will recover. Who will recover. Who will not recover.

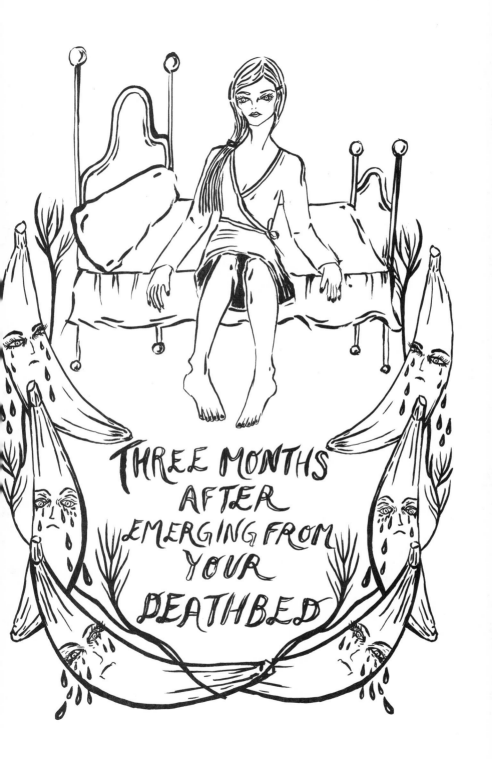

THREE MONTHS AFTER emerging from your deathbed, you may find that you wonder why you bothered. You will have just survived a remarkable medical feat, perhaps with no explanation, and you are expected to be filled with gratitude. You try. Many days, you shed tears of relief, or unprocessed fear. On other days, you cry because for however long—three months, maybe—you had wished yourself off your deathbed under the unshakable belief that something bigger and better was awaiting you. Now you see that it was not. What terrifies you most after emerging from your deathbed is realizing how little difference your death would have made, how little difference it didn't end up making after all.

You may become angry with yourself; in fact, you will become angry with yourself, for good reason. You are an ungrateful shit to have survived such trauma and emerge from it with only malaise. How dare you take this hard-earned gift of life and treat it so unkindly? When you watched movies on your deathbed, which you did quite often, and characters said unthoughtful things about the meaninglessness of life or ending it all, you would cringe or yell or cry. Remembering a friend's casual joke about wishing she were dead on the day your doctor gave you bad news about your heart function still makes you wince. Now you say such things yourself. Your anger compounds: for you are not only an ingrate, you are also a hypocrite.

Perhaps you should have died; perhaps you should die now because you are so horrible.

At the three-month mark, perhaps you will remember how you used to cope with your always precarious future, before it came under direct threat. You may recall, too, how you used to make plans with friends to ward off rare stretches of unstructured days, how you enjoyed the company, the conversations that moved freely from topic to topic. Even remembering that you used to do this is a sign that your enthusiasms are returning. You also used to apply for things: opportunities, awards, jobs. You did this to exercise intellectual promiscuity. It felt expansive. You used to plan trips, some you would not even take. And work! You used to love it, although you cannot now remember why. You used to read things that had nothing to do with your immediate physical survival, or eat foods because they seemed interesting and not because they contained healthy elements your kidneys or muscle tissue could not do without. You will remember this and begin to wonder if you will ever regain the excess of energy required to do it again. To make plans as if you had all the time in the world, as if you could follow through with them. You had forgotten what it was like to operate without a deadline, or that it was possible to do so.

Your friends, especially if they are middle-aged, will say: *Oh, I know. What is the point? I feel exactly the same way. It is the politics/the season/climate change/the economy.* You will say, *Yes, but also I almost died.* And they will say, *Oh yeah. I'm glad you're feeling better now.* You will feel disappointed by this, although it is unclear why. You completely understand why your friends would be bored by your recent medical drama. You, too, are bored of it. You also understand that they are middle-aged, and you are middle-aged, and maybe really it is a phase of the life you just saved that you cannot escape: malaise. Maybe the thing about emerging from your deathbed is that it ended up mattering so little, your survival, that you are still beholden to the same whims and extravagances that fill regular people's lives. Maybe your life, in fact, is just like everyone else's, deathbed or no.

You might visit a therapist. If you had been seeing a therapist while on your deathbed, the therapist will remind you that you have made remarkable progress, will exclaim that just so many weeks ago you did not know if you could make plans to see friends or if you should bother buying groceries. The therapist will remind you that the increase in energy required to meet all the minimum daily upkeep tasks you now perform to stay alive displays an enthusiasm unprecedented in recent days; that you can even consider taking a long view at this time and pondering the worth of it all shows great progress over a few short months earlier. The therapist will ask you to refrain from expressing an excess of criticism of your life right now. Unfortunately, the therapist will have no idea who you are, really, no idea what you were like before the deathbed, no idea that a little over so many months ago, you could never have invited such feel-good meaninglessness into your life. It is not an excess of bitterness you sling in the therapist's direction, but a real and relevant question: If I survived all this, why?

In other words, you do all the things at the three-month mark that indicate emotional healing. You take steps to consider and improve your worldview. (That the worldview itself does not improve seems to bother only you:

everyone else is thrilled by it.) You maintain a daily regimen of physical health, however minimal. (Although privately you calculate its cost and purpose.) That you get out of bed at all seems enough for everyone around you. Was it ever enough before? The people congratulating you now have attended your book-release parties, your art openings, your award ceremonies, your graduation events. Were they faking it then, by saying that they always knew you were capable of greatness? Or are they faking it now, by telling you that they are just happy you are alive?

One day, three months after you emerge from your deathbed, a friend will invite you to sushi. He once abandoned you at a moment of great need. He had failed to recognize the danger you were in while you were on your deathbed, and remained wrapped up in his own drama when you needed him to concentrate fully on yours. But it is much easier to forgive him for these transgressions than to forgive yourself for having become sick. So you agree to meet him and to have lunch with him.

As you sit down to order, you will remember about sushi. It will be the first time in many months that you have considered the experience of eating raw and perfectly prepared seafood: The coldness of it. The extraterrestrial aroma and sharp, clear colors. The perfect alarm of wasabi and the clean, earthy warmth of long-grain rice. The delightful nuance of flavors in fresh-caught fish from different parts of the world, subtly complemented with saltiness, tanginess, sweetness. You have not even ordered yet, but looking at the menu will stir something in you. The restaurant will be busy, and the couple sitting next to you appear to be on an awkward first date. They have come to the best sushi restaurant in one of the best sushi cities in the world, and you will be reminded about all the minor life choices that it took for you to even know about this place: how you found yourself living with your friend in an art residency on the East Coast, how you became close under unlikely circumstances and then, under even more unlikely circumstances, ended up visiting him on the opposite end of the country on a fairly consistent basis. You weren't sure whether or not you would ever actually be friends, or who this person even was, until one day he put a banana in his pocket as you were piling into a car to attend a group function and he sat next to you. You made a joke: *Is that a banana in your pocket or are you just happy to see me?* The joke then became something else, not about erections or men being inappropriate or fruits that look like penises or even an unspoken attraction between you two, but a joke about carrying bananas around town because in the end that was the funniest part: that someone might ever, for any reason, be carrying a banana around in their pocket.

You will be reminded of the hilarity of the banana joke while reading the menu, which will contain everything you have ever wanted to eat in that moment, and there it is, open in front of you. In a list. You can tally how many of each piece of sushi you want and they will bring it to you, and the astonishment of this catches you at the base of your throat, somewhere above your left lung. You are overwhelmed with gratitude, shaking with it. You will order everything, you actually will, but there is a particular thing that you like there that combines deep-fried rice and spicy tuna, and when it arrives and you take a bite of it you can feel the soft fish and the sharpness of the chili peppers and the hard, sweet crunch of the rice. You will be eating across the table from your friend, next to a couple on a first date that doesn't seem to be going very well, in a crowded restaurant, but you will also be crying. Giant tears will be dropping from your eyes at the sheer overwhelming wonder of this exact moment and how lucky you are to experience it.

Then—as does everything, eventually—the moment will pass. When you glance down at the table, your tears are there, still pooled. Partially to distract your friend from your tears, but also because it is true, you will ask your friend, "You know what fucking sucks?"

He will look at you blankly. He has just been expressing concern about his own life, and you are being a dick by interrupting him and averting the attention to yourself. But you could not fucking care less because you are alive and you have thought of something true to say.

"One thing that fucking sucks is thinking you're going to die every day for three months." You will say this venomously, like how people exaggerate meaningless things for the sake of comedy. Except here there is no exaggeration, no joke.

Your friend will burst out laughing anyway. He has a loud laugh, the laugh of a man who is secure in the world, a comforting laugh. The entire restaurant will respond to his laughter; some people will smile along with him. Then you laugh too. You had forgotten about laughing the way you had forgotten about sushi. You laugh hard and long. Your laugh is frenetic, contagious. It always has been; it has just been dormant. Hearing it now makes others laugh too. Soon everyone in the whole restaurant is happy, including the couple sitting next to you, and no one realizes that this is because you did not die. You had forgotten how easy it is to make people happy, how easy it is to be happy yourself.

"That shit is the worst," you will say to your friend, before picking up your chopsticks to begin eating again. You will roll your eyes for emphasis. You will both laugh again because it is true.

Then it will be over. You will no longer be someone who has just emerged from a deathbed. You will just be an alive person, whole again, living your life.

PUBLICATION CREDITS

I am deeply indebted to the teams who published early drafts of the work included in this volume. A version of "Massacre on Veng Sreng Street" appeared in the *Los Angeles Review of Books Quarterly* in 2014, and an early version of "The Shameful Legacy (and Secret Promise) of the Sanitary Napkin Disposal Bag" was published that same year in *The Baffler*. "Tips, Gags, and Jokes for Girls in Captivity" appeared in 2020 as a Pressing Concern Book Mark. Sections of "Women" appeared in 2013 on the now-defunct *The Blog Is Coming from Inside the House*. A portion of an earlier version of "Model Employee" was published in *Talking Points Memo* in 2015. Parts of "Consumpcyon" first appeared in the *Women's Review of Books* in 2016. "Fake Snake Oil" was first published in *The State* in 2012. "On Leaving the Birthplace of Standard Time" was written for the Miss Spoken Reading Series at the Gallery Cabaret in Chicago, and the version from the first edition of this book appeared in *The Believer* in 2017. Early versions of "The Presence of No Present" and "Fucking Cancer" formed the basis of a 2015 performance lecture given at the University of Illinois at Chicago's Gallery 400. A portion of the former essay was also used to create a sound art piece for SPACES in Cleveland, Ohio, in 2016. An early version of "The Metaphysics of Compost" was published on the Write A House blog in 2016. Sections of "Normative Bodies, Unusual Tastes" were originally published in the introduction to the first edition of *Body Horror* in 2017.

NOTES

Massacre on Veng Sreng Street

1. Human Rights Watch, "Cambodia: Hun Sen and His Abusive Generals," October 22, 2020, https://www.hrw.org/news/2020/10/22/cambodia-hun-sen-and-his-abusive-generals.

2. United States Environmental Protection Agency, "National Overview: Facts and Figures on Materials, Wastes and Recycling," updated July 31, 2022, https://www.epa.gov/facts-and-figures-about-materials-waste-and-recycling/national-overview-facts-and-figures-materials.

The Shameful Legacy (and Secret Promise) of the Sanitary Napkin Disposal Bag

1. For more on this, see Vern L. Bullough, "Merchandising the Sanitary Napkin: Lillian Gilbreth's 1927 Survey," *Signs: Journal of Women in Culture and Society* 10, no. 3 (Spring 1985): 615–27.

2. Clara Guibourg and Nassos Stylianou, "Why are so few women inventors named on patents?," BBC News, October 2, 2019, https://www.bbc.com/news/technology-49843990.

3. Jennifer Hunt, Jean-Philippe Garant, Hannah Herman, and David J. Munroe, "Why Don't Women Patent?" (working paper, National Bureau of Economic Research, March 2012), http://www.nber.org/papers/w17888?ntw.

4. Jessica Milli, Barbara Gault, Emma Williams-Baron, Jenny Xia, and Meika Berlan, "The Gender Patenting Gap," Institute for Women's Policy Research, July 2016, https://iwpr.org/wp-content/uploads/2020/12/C441_Gender-Patenting-Gap_BP-1.pdf.

5. National Women's Law Center, "The Wage Gap Is Stagnant in Last Decade," September 2012, https://nwlc.org/wp-content/uploads/2015/08/wage_gap_is_stagnant_2013_1.pdf.

6. Bryce Covert, "Women Aren't Held Back By an Ambition Gap. They're Just Held Back," *Forbes*, November 14, 2012, http://www.forbes.com/sites/brycecovert/2012/11/14/

women-arent-held-back-by-an-ambition-gap-theyre-just-held-back/.

7. Claire Ewing-Nelson and Jasmine Tucker, "A Year into the Pandemic, Women Are Still Short Nearly 5.1 Million Jobs," National Women's Law Center, March 5, 2021, https://nwlc.org/resource/feb-jobs-2021/.

8. National Women's Business Council, *Intellectual Property and Women Entrepreneurs: Quantitative Analysis*, 2012, https://cdn.www.nwbc.gov/wp-content/uploads/2018/02/27192725/Qualitative-Analysis-Intellectual-Property-Women-Entrepreneurs-Part-1.pdf.

9. Kyle Jensen, Balázs Kovács, and Olav Sorenson, "Gender differences in obtaining and maintaining patent rights," *Nature Biotechnology* 36, no. 4 (April 2018): 307–9, https://www.nature.com/articles/nbt.4120.epdf.

10. Ann Germanow, "The Most Hazardous Spot in Women's Restrooms," Building Services Management, 2009, http://www.bsmmag.com/Main/Articles/2009/09/FeminineCareProductDisposal.htm. Interestingly, the original letter has disappeared since I first published this piece with *The Baffler* in June 2014, although it was archived in February 2012 by the Internet Archive, retrieved August 26, 2022: https://web.archive.org/web/20120228181704/http://www.bsmmag.com/Main/Articles/2009/09/Feminine%20Care%20Product%20Disposal.htm.

11. These are tallied by way of Google Patents; gender was determined by name and further online investigation. Both processes are somewhat flawed.

Women

1. For the remainder of this essay, I will use the term *misogyny* to refer to all gender-based violence afflicting folks outside the strictly masculine end of the gender spectrum. I have no wish to erase trans and nonbinary folks, not even in language, but it is the term under consideration in the works of the artists I address here. I also desire the language that I use to reflect the world as I genuinely experience it, and my experience suggests that femininity in any degree, regardless of the gender identity of the performer, is the real target of misogyny. (I remain open to correction on this point.)

2. Nicolas Rapold, "Hard Life for a von Trier Woman, Again," *New York Times*, February 28, 2014, https://www.nytimes.com/2014/03/02/movies/hard-life-for-a-von-trier-woman-again.html.

3. Virginie Despentes, *King Kong Theory*, trans. Frank Wynne (New York: Farrar, Straus and Giroux, 2021), 28.

4. Despentes, 38.

5. Despentes, 40.

6. Roger Ebert, "*I Spit on Your Grave*," RogerEbert.com, July 16, 1980, retrieved August 26, 2022, http://www.rogerebert. com/reviews/i-spit-on-your-grave-1980. Originally published in the *Chicago Sun-Times*.

7. Carol J. Clover, *Men, Women, and Chain Saws: Gender in the Modern Horror Film* (Princeton, NJ: Princeton University Press, 1992), 115.

8. Despentes, 39.

9. Despentes, 44.

Model Employee

1. Jennifer Sky, "Does Fashion Week Exploit Teen Models?" *Daily Beast*, last modified July 12, 2017, http://www. thedailybeast.com/articles/2014/09/14/does-fashion-week-exploit-teen-models.html.

2. Jennifer Sky, "Jennifer Sky, Fashion Week and Exploitation," *Guernica*, September 10, 2012, https://www. guernicamag.com/daily/jennifer-sky-fashion-week-and-exploitation/.

3. The Model Alliance, "Models' Bill of Rights," September 5, 2015, Wayback Machine, accessed October 28, 2022, https:// web.archive.org/web/20150905052900/http:/modelalliance. org/models-bill-of-rights.

4. This text was from a pop-up ad on the Model Alliance website circa 2015, still live as of October 28, 2016, at http:// modelalliance.org, although as of August 26, 2022, it no longer appears there, as the calendar has been discontinued.

5. Eugene Whong, "Cambodia Increases Minimum Wage to $200 a Month," Radio Free Asia, September 21, 2022, https:// www.rfa.org/english/news/cambodia/minimum_wage-09212022172817.html.

6. Abby Edge and Sheng Lu, "How Will EU Trade Curb Affect Cambodia's Apparel Industry?" Just Style, June 16, 2020, https://www.just-style.com/analysis/how-will-eu-trade-curb-affect-cambodias-apparel-industry/.

7. Better Factories Cambodia, "Twenty First Synthesis Report on Working Conditions in Cambodia's Garment Sector," International Labour Organization, October 31, 2008, https:// www.ohchr.org/sites/default/files/lib-docs/HRBodies/UPR/

Documents/Session6/KH/UNCT_KHM_UPRS06_2009_
document7.pdf.

8. CARE Australia, "Women in Cambodia's Garment Industry: Their Work, Their Safety," report taken from CARE study *"I know I cannot quit." The Prevalence and Productivity Cost of Sexual Harassment to the Cambodian Garment Industry*, March 2017, https://www.care.org.au/wp-content/uploads/2017/04/SHCS_Brief-Women-Cambodia-Garment-Industry-March-2017_CA.pdf.

9. Laura Babbit, Drusilla Brown, and Ana Antolin, "Sexual Harassment: Causes and Remediation, Evidence from Better Factories Cambodia," International Labour Organization, September 2020, https://betterwork.org/wp-content/uploads/2020/10/DP-38-Sexual-harassment-causes-and-remediation-BFC.pdf.

10. Model Alliance, "2012 Industry Survey Report," accessed October 28, 2022, https://www.modelalliance.org/published.

11. "Occupational Outlook Handbook: Models," US Bureau of Labor Statistics, last modified September 8, 2021, https://www.bls.gov/ooh/sales/models.htm.

12. For my in-depth analysis: Anne Elizabeth Moore, "The Fashion Industry's Perfect Storm: Collapsing Workers and Hyperactive Buyers," *Truthout*, April 4, 2012, http://truth-out.org/news/item/8307-the-fashion-industrys-perfect-storm-collapsing-workers-and-hyperactive-buyers.

13. Sara Ziff, "Yes, you should feel bad for models: we're being told to diet—or go broke," *The Guardian*, September 9, 2014, http://www.theguardian.com/commentisfree/2014/sep/09/models-diet-go-broke-modeling-industry?CMP=twt_gu.

14. Jennifer Sky, "Protect Children in the Fashion Industry from Exploitation," YouTube, February 3, 2014, https://www.youtube.com/watch?v=kKJ99GhOUN0.

15. For more on these fascinating denationalized zones, see my comic with Melissa Mendes: Anne Elizabeth Moore and Melissa Mendes, "Ladydrawers—Zoned: The Mysterious 'Foreign' Outposts Inside the USA," *Truthout*, November 12, 2013, http://truth-out.org/opinion/item/19977-ladydrawers-zoned (also included in my 2016 book *Threadbare: Clothes, Sex & Trafficking*). See also Dara Orenstein, *Out of Stock: The Warehouse in the History of Capitalism* (Chicago: The University of Chicago Press, 2019).

16. This rose dramatically by the 2015 report, when $13.23

328

was listed as the mean hourly pay for models. Unfortunately, the living wage in New York rose just as dramatically, to $14.52, which narrows the gap between earnings and living wage only slightly.

17. Check MIT's Living Wage Calculator, retrieved August 26, 2022: http://livingwage.mit.edu/states/36.

18. Living wage in Mexico and Bangladesh for 2022 from Global Living Wage Coalition, *Living Wage Update Report: Michoacán, Mexico, 2022*, April 5, 2022, https:// globallivingwage.org/wp-content/uploads/2020/10/ Updatereport_Mexico_2022_RAMA_final.pdf, and "Living Wage for Dhaka City, Bangladesh," Global Living Wage Coalition, accessed July 26, 2022, https://www. globallivingwage.org/living-wage-benchmarks/urban-bangladesh/, respectively. Average monthly wages for 2022 garment-factory workers in Mexico from "Fashion and Apparel Average Salaries in Mexico 2022," Salary Explorer, accessed July 26, 2022, http://www.salaryexplorer.com/salary-survey. php?loc=139&loctype=1&job=25&jobtype=1#:~:text=A%20 person%20working%20in%20Fashion%20and%20 Apparel%20in%20Mexico%20typically,actual%20 maximum%20salary%20is%20higher, and in Bangladesh from Dave Lesser, "Garment Worker Diaries Update in Bangladesh through May 2022," Garment Worker Diaries, July 7, 2022, https://workerdiaries.org/garment-worker-diaries-update-in-bangladesh-through-may-2022/#:~:text=78%25%20 of%20all%20garment%20workers,median%20salary%20 amount%20of%20Tk.

19. Worker Rights Consortium, *Stealing from the Poor: Wage Theft in the Haitian Garment Industry*, October 15, 2013, https://www.workersrights.org/research-report/stealing-from-the-poor-wage-theft-in-the-haitian-apparel-industry/.

20. "About," Vetan Chori Band Karo / Campaign to stop wage theft, accessed August 26, 2022, http:// vetanchoribandkaro.wordpress.com/about-2/.

21. Dave Jamieson, "Walmart Warehouse Contractor To Pay $21 Million To Settle Wage Theft Allegations," last modified May 14, 2014, https://www.huffpost.com/entry/walmart-warehouse-wage-theft_n_5324021.

22. Admittedly, this is only one in a sea of hundreds or thousands of class-action lawsuits filed against Forever 21, distinguishable only by its association with a particular warehouse. Shan Li, "Forever 21 employees file class action

lawsuit," *Los Angeles Times*, January 19, 2012, http://articles.latimes.com/2012/jan/19/business/la-fi-mo-forever-21-lawsuit-20120119.

23. "Fashion brands fail to address pandemic-era wage theft in Cambodia," Clean Clothes Campaign, July 14, 2021, https://cleanclothes.org/news/2021/fashion-brands-fail-to-address-pandemic-era-wage-theft-in-cambodia.

24. Ziff, "Yes, you should feel bad for models."

25. Jenna Sauers, "Fashion Week's Models Are Getting Whiter," *Jezebel*, February 18, 2013, http://jezebel.com/5985110/new-york-fashion-weeks-models-are-getting-whiter.

26. Jessica Andrews, "Despite Gains, the Fall 2016 Runways Were Still Less Than 25 Percent Diverse (Report)," *Fashion Spot*, March 16, 2016, http://www.thefashionspot.com/runway-news/685109-runway-diversity-report-fall-2016/.

27. Vanessa Friedman, Salamishah Tillet, Elizabeth Paton, Jessica Testa, and Evan Nicole Brown, "The Fashion World Promised More Diversity. Here's What We Found," *New York Times*, March 4, 2021, https://www.nytimes.com/2021/03/04/style/Black-representation-fashion.html.

Horror Autotoxicus

1. *Proto*, "The Salvarsan Wars," May 3, 2010, http://protomag.com/articles/paul-ehrlich-and-the-salvarsan-wars.

2. Ernst Bäumler, *Paul Ehrlich: Scientist for Life*, trans. Grant Edwards (New York: Holmes & Meier, 1984), 200.

3. Bäumler, *Paul Ehrlich*, 200.

4. Amanda Yarnell, "Salvarsan: Purpose Antisyphilitic," *Chemical & Engineering News*, June 20, 2005, https://cen.acs.org/articles/83/i25/Salvarsan.html.

5. Adalimimab's mortality rates have since been scrubbed from Medpage Today's site, but were available here under the heading "Adalimimab" on May 31, 2019: https://www.medpagetoday.org/meetingcoverage/eular/20766?vpass=1.

6. See Ernst Bäumler's *Paul Ehrlich* for an excellent description of these events.

7. "Pinkus Family Genealogy," accessed July 29, 2022, http://freepages.rootsweb.com/~prohel/genealogy/names/pinkus/pinkus.html.

8. Bäumler, *Paul Ehrlich*, 226.

9. "How did Public Opinion About Entering World War II Change Between 1939 and 1941?" United States Holocaust

Memorial Museum, accessed August 16, 2022, https://exhibitions.ushmm.org/americans-and-the-holocaust/us-public-opinion-world-war-II-1939-1941.

10. "Autoimmunity may be rising in the United States," National Institutes of Health, April 8, 2020, https://www.nih.gov/news-events/news-releases/autoimmunity-may-be-rising-united-states.

11. Martha Marquardt, *Paul Ehrlich* (New York, Schuman: 1951), 89–90.

12. Quoted in Bäumler, *Paul Ehrlich*, 20.

13. Quoted in Bäumler, *Paul Ehrlich*, 20.

14. Irvine Loudon, "Deaths in Childbed from the Eighteenth Century to 1935," *Medical History* 30, no. 1 (1986): 1–41, https://pubmed.ncbi.nlm.nih.gov/3511335/.

Consumpcyon

1. This and all other Atwood quotations come from the 1999 edition of *The Edible Woman*, published by McClelland & Stewart in Toronto.

2. Millicent Bell, "The Girl on the Wedding Cake," *New York Times*, October 18, 1970, https://www.nytimes.com/books/00/09/03/specials/atwood-edible.html.

3. Michael Pollan, *The Omnivore's Dilemma: A Natural History of Four Meals* (New York: Penguin Books, 2007), 16.

4. Rachel, "Laying off the pizza for a while," *My Life with IBS*, December 2, 2009, http://ibsrachel.blogspot.com/2009/12/laying-off-pizza-for-while.html.

5. National Institute of Environmental Health Sciences, "Autoimmune Diseases," updated May 31, 2022, https://www.niehs.nih.gov/health/topics/conditions/autoimmune/index.cfm.

6. National Institutes of Health: The Autoimmune Diseases Coordinating Committee, "Progress in Autoimmune Diseases Research: Report to Congress," US Department of Health and Human Services, March 2005, https://www.niaid.nih.gov/sites/default/files/adccfinal.pdf.

7. Rachel, "Wedding Series: In-Laws," *My Life with IBS*, January 9, 2014, http://ibsrachel.blogspot.com/2014/01/wedding-series-in-laws.html.

8. Diane E. Hoffmann and Anita J. Tarzian, "The Girl Who Cried Pain: A Bias Against Women in the Treatment of Pain," *Journal of Law, Medicine and Ethics* 29 (2001): 13–27, https://papers.ssrn.com/sol3/papers.cfm?abstract_id=383803.

9. Mary Jo DiLonardo, "Why do doctors take women's pain less seriously?" *Mother Nature Network*, October 23, 2015, accessed November 1, 2016, http://www.mnn.com/health/fitness-well-being/stories/why-do-doctors-take-womens-pain-less-seriously, although the article has been scrubbed from the new site, *Treehugger*.

10. Those invested in mainstream feminism could and should ask why autoimmune disease is not an issue of concern on the level of reproductive health, but I won't spoil the fun for you by explaining it here.

11. Aaron Lerner and Torsten Matthias, "Changes in intestinal tight junction permeability associated with industrial food additives explain the rising incidence of autoimmune disease," *Autoimmunity Reviews* 14, no. 6 (June 2015): 479–89, https://www.sciencedirect.com/science/article/pii/S1568997215000245?via%3Dihub.

12. The Times Editorial Board, "Editorial: Food labels and the trouble with trade deals," *Los Angeles Times*, May 20, 2015, http://www.latimes.com/opinion/editorials/la-ed-food-labels-20150520-story.html.

13. *The Omnivore's Dilemma*, 113.

14. As quoted in Susan Sontag, *Illness as Metaphor and AIDS and Its Metaphors* (New York: Picador, 2001) 9.

15. Jean M. Lawrence et al., "Trends in Prevalence of Type 1 and Type 2 Diabetes in Children and Adolescents in the US, 2001–2017," *JAMA* 326, no. 8 (August 24, 2021): 717–27, https://jamanetwork.com/journals/jama/fullarticle/2783420.

Fake Snake Oil

1. Russel Heimlich, "Wikipedia Users," Pew Research Center, January 13, 2011, https://www.pewresearch.org/fact-tank/2011/01/13/wikipedia-users/.

2. J. Frank Dobie, *Rattlesnakes: The Age-Old Feud between Snake and Man!* (Austin: University of Texas Press, 1982), 75.

3. Lisa Hix, "How Snake Oil Got a Bad Rap (Hint: It Wasn't the Snakes' Fault)," Collectors Weekly, May 20, 2011, https://www.collectorsweekly.com/articles/how-snake-oil-got-a-bad-rap/.

4. Michelle Ferranti, "An Odor of Racism: Vaginal Deodorants in African-American Beauty Culture and Advertising," *Advertising & Society Review* 11, no. 4 (2011), https://doi.org/10.1353/asr.2011.0003.

5. Thomas Jefferson, *Notes on the State of Virginia*, PDF (Sam Houston State University), accessed October 29, 2022,

https://www.shsu.edu/~jll004/163_spring09/jefferson_
race.pdf.

6. Bettina Hitzer, "The Odor of Disgust: Contemplating
the Dark Side of 20th-Century Cancer History," *Emotion
Review* 12, no. 3 (February 28, 2020): 156–67, https://journals.
sagepub.com/doi/10.1177/1754073919897293.

On Leaving the Birthplace of Standard Time

1. Maria R. Traska, "Route 66 history: welcoming Standard
Time and time zones," *The Curious Traveler's Guide to
Route 66 in Metro Chicago*, November 4, 2014, https://
curioustraveler66.wordpress.com/2014/11/04/route-66-
history-welcoming-standard-time-and-time-zones/.

2. It sits approximately twenty-three blocks south and
twelve blocks east of where I first delivered this piece on the
Near North Side in Chicago, a distance it takes me an hour and
a half to cross when I decide to test it.

Cultural Imperative

1. It may be interesting that my actual class status changed
at this time: family relationships disintegrated, so I had
no economic foundation to rely on, concurrent with the
disintegration of my health, although that wouldn't become
evident for a few more years. I looked the part, in other words,
but it was already evident to me that the way I was read had
little to do with the resources I had access to.

2. Madhavi Sunder, *From Goods to a Good Life: Intellectual
Property and Global Justice* (New Haven, CT: Yale University
Press, 2012), 23.

3. Jennifer Hunt, Jean-Philippe Garant, Hannah Herman,
and David J. Munroe, "Why Don't Women Patent?" (working
paper, National Bureau of Economic Research, Cambridge, MA,
March 2012), https://www.nber.org/papers/w17888.

4. World Intellectual Property Organization, "Gender
Equality, Diversity and Intellectual Property," accessed
October 29, 2022, https://www.wipo.int/women-and-ip/en/.

5. Quoted in *Diamond v. Chakrabarty*, 447 U.S. 303, 100
S.Ct. 2204, 65 L.Ed.2d 144 (1980), https://h2o.law.harvard.
edu/collages/14582.

6. All Vandana Shiva quotations come from *Protect
or Plunder?: Understanding Intellectual Property Rights*
(London: Zed Books, 2001), originally published as *Patents:
Myths and Reality* (New Delhi: Penguin Books, 2001).

7. Shiva, 17.

8. Sunder, *From Goods to a Good Life*, 32.

The Presence of No Present

1. Alison Kafer, *Feminist, Queer, Crip* (Bloomington: Indiana University Press, 2013), 33.

Normative Bodies, Unusual Tastes

1. Martha M. Lauzen, "The Celluloid Ceiling in a Pandemic Year: Employment of Women on the Top U.S. Films of 2021," Center for the Study of Women in Television and Film, accessed October 29, 2022, https://womenintvfilm.sdsu.edu/wp-content/uploads/2022/01/2021-Celluloid-Ceiling-Report.pdf.

2. Martha M. Lauzen, "Living Archive: The Celluloid Ceiling Documenting Two Decades of Women's Employment in Film," Center for the Study of Women in Television and Film, accessed October 29, 2022, https://womenintvfilm.sdsu.edu/wp-content/uploads/2020/12/2020_Living_Archive_Report.pdf.

3. The cartoonist Gabrielle Gamboa and I made a comic to illustrate some data we'd pulled during the #31HorrorFilms31Days Twitter challenge hosted at the time by Daniel Kraus at *Booklist*. Hashtag contributors are urged to watch a film every day in October and then tweet a review/summary. In 2012, a few of us (Rob Kirby's contributions stand out, alongside the above participants) further took note of basic demographic data on cast and crew, as well as key plot points. Further content analysis I performed on my own because I secretly love doing math. Anne Elizabeth Moore and Gabrielle Gamboa, "The truly scary politics of horror movies," *Salon*, October 29, 2013, http://www.salon.com/2013/10/29/the_truly_scary_politics_of_horror_movies/.

4. In her long-running comic strip, *Dykes to Watch Out For*, Alison Bechdel has two characters in a strip from 1985 discussing the minimal criteria for attending a film: that it include at least two female characters talking to each other about something besides a man. Even Bechdel was surprised, years later, to discover it still had currency. "I feel a little bit sheepish about the whole thing, because it's not like I invented this test or said, 'This is the Bechdel Test.' It somehow has gotten attributed to me over the years. . . . It's this weird thing.

People actually use it to analyze films to see whether or not they pass that test," Bechdel told NPR's Terry Gross on *Fresh Air*. (For the record, Bechdel credits her friend Liz Wallace with these rules and would prefer it be called the Bechdel-Wallace Test.)

5. "Campus Sexual Violence: Statistics," Rape, Abuse & Incest National Network, accessed October 11, 2022, https://www.rainn.org/statistics/campus-sexual-violence.

6. Hannah Ellis-Petersen, "Tom Six: 'In 100 years people will still be talking about my human centipede films,'" *The Guardian*, July 2, 2015, https://www.theguardian.com/film/2015/jul/02/human-centipede-director-tom-six-i-have-this-very-sick-imagination.

7. Rich Juzwiak, "'I Don't Like Human Beings': A Chat with *The Human Centipede*'s Tom Six," *Defamer*, May 21, 2015, http://defamer.gawker.com/i-dont-like-human-beings-a-chat-with-the-human-centi-1706049658.

8. Michael Guillen, "*Deadgirl*—Interview with Gadi Harel," ScreenAnarchy, March 8, 2009, http://screenanarchy.com/2009/03/deadgirlinterview-with-gadi-harel.html.

9. *Deadgirl*, in truth, does offer an interesting and knowing view on misogyny, for a film about a group of young men finding a young woman and mutilating her is, fundamentally, about what culture suggests is acceptable for men to do to women's bodies. It is, however, a far cry from being a feminist film, in content or in production.

10. I suspect this has so far kept most filmmakers from making body-horror films about trans and nonbinary individuals, relying overmuch on the questionable notion that stripping away gender equates to a loss of personhood.

The Metaphysics of Compost

1. "An Organic Theory of Composting," *Los Angeles Times*, December 31, 1989, http://articles.latimes.com/1989-12-31/opinion/op-464_1_compost-pile.

2. Kim Q. Hall, "Toward a Queer Crip Feminist Politics of Food," *philoSOPHIA: A Journal of Continental Feminism* 4, no. 2 (Summer 2014): 177–96, http://www.academia.edu/7703970/Toward_a_Queer_Crip_Feminist_Politics_of_Food.

3. Hall, 179.

4. Hall, 179.

Fucking Cancer

1. Susan Sontag, *Illness as Metaphor and AIDS and Its Metaphors* (New York: Picador, 2001), 3. This and all other Sontag quotations are taken from this edition.

2. Sontag, 99.

3. Sontag, 101.

4. This and the following quotations appear in Arthur M. Silverstein, "Autoimmunity *versus horror autotoxicus*: The struggle for recognition," *Nature Immunology* 2 (2001): 279–81, http://www.nature.com/ni/journal/v2/n4/full/ni0401_279.html.

5. Sontag, 99.

6. American Autoimmune Related Diseases Association, "1-in-5 Brochure," 2019, https://autoimmune.org/wp-content/uploads/2019/12/1-in-5-Brochure.pdf.

7. According to the World Cancer Research Fund, online at http://wcrf.org.

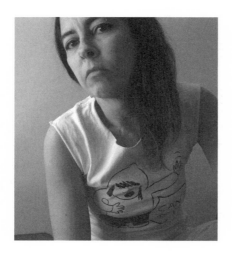

ANNE ELIZABETH MOORE is the author of *Unmarketable*, the Eisner Award–winning *Sweet Little Cunt*, *Gentrifier*, which was an NPR Best Book of the Year, and others. She is the founding editor of *The Best American Comics* and the former editor of *Punk Planet*, *The Comics Journal*, and the *Chicago Reader*. She has written for *The Guardian*, *The Baffler*, and *The Onion*. Moore is a Fulbright Senior Scholar and a former Mackey Chair in Creative Writing at Beloit College, and has received support for her work from the National Endowment for the Arts, the Corporation of Yaddo, and the New York State Council on the Arts. She currently teaches at the School of Visual Arts and lives in New York with two ineffective feline personal assistants.

The Feminist Press publishes books that
ignite movements and social transformation.
Celebrating our legacy, we lift up insurgent
and marginalized voices from around the
world to build a more just future.

See our complete list of books at
feministpress.org

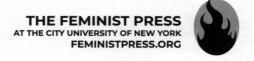

THE FEMINIST PRESS
AT THE CITY UNIVERSITY OF NEW YORK
FEMINISTPRESS.ORG